Studying a Study and
Testing a Test

HOW TO
READ THE
MEDICAL
LITERATURE

Studying a Study and
Testing a Test

HOW TO
READ THE
MEDICAL
LITERATURE

Richard K. Riegelman, M.D., M.P.H.

Assistant Professor, Department of Health Care Sciences and Department of Medicine, The George Washington University Medical Center, Washington, D.C.; Attending Physician, The George Washington University Hospital, Washington, D.C.

Little, Brown and Company, Boston

Preface

Today's practicing clinicians are confronted with an enormous number of journal articles, a virtual deluge of data, and with the dilemma of how best to evaluate this information and incorporate it into their clinical practices. In order to cope with the need to keep up with the current findings of medical science, clinicians can do one of two things: they can simply memorize information, thereby adopting unquestioningly either the latest innovation or the newest technology; or they can learn how to use the techniques that are available for a more critical, and ultimately more useful, reading of the medical literature.

Unfortunately, one particular fallacy concerning the nature of scientific research often deters critical analysis. The idea has taken hold that common sense can make no contribution and that only the experts can critique the reports of medical research, an idea that robs clinicians of their most powerful prerogative—the ability to decide for themselves. This self-study, active-participation book was written to dispel this fallacy and to show clinicians how to read the medical literature thoughtfully and efficiently. The techniques that will be described do not require a specialized knowledge since they are based on the systematic use of clinical common sense.

The application of a science or a technology to any area of inquiry, however, requires the initial understanding of its assumptions, implications, and limitations. For this reason, statistical concepts are presented here, and their implications and assumptions are defined, but there is no undue emphasis on carrying out statistical manipulations. Instead, the emphasis is placed on clarifying the question that is being asked by a study, on determining whether a correct statistical test is being used, and on understanding the meaning of the results.

Any useful approach to reading the medical literature must build on, and be compatible with, clinical training. In the differential diagnosis approach to clinical problems, an organized, structured framework helps clinicians to think through a problem rapidly. Similarly, the reader of this book is given a uniform framework on which to build a critique of any research article. A checklist of questions for the reader to ask when evaluating a study also helps to develop a systematic approach that will speed up the process of analyzing articles.

Much as in learning to perform a physical examination, the reader's attention is directed initially to the individual components of the process. Capsule summaries of hypothetical journal articles, each focused on a particular type of error, help to illustrate and crystallize the complementary parts of analysis. The time spent in learning the basic principles pays off in ability to comprehend more quickly the meaning and the limitations of any study one encounters.

The case-study method used here, which is similar to ward training or clinical/pathological conferences, provides the active "hands-on" training needed to internalize the concepts and gain proficiency in using them. At the end of each section are flaw-catching exercises—simulated articles fraught with a variety of errors—that provide practice in applying the uniform framework. A sample critique of each flaw-catching exercise allows readers to evaluate the progress they are making in analyzing the material. A flowsheet, which summarizes the various statistical methods, guides the reader through the steps involved in statistical thinking. As in clinical training, the goal is an organized analysis of the data that will provide a basis for decision-making.

The immediate aim of this book is to help clinicians assess the degree and type of uncertainty that exist in a particular piece of medical research, since the constraints on most medical research often result in data that are inconclusive. It must be stressed, however, that studies that are less than ideal do not necessarily invalidate research or relieve clinicians of their responsibility to draw clinical conclusions.

The overall objective is for clinicians to learn the kinds of questions that statistics can answer as well as the kinds of questions they must answer for themselves. Clinicians who can critically read the medical literature, and understand and accept the uncertainty that exists, are better able to draw meaningful conclusions that will help them to integrate the results of medical research into their clinical practices.

R.K.R.

Acknowledgments

The professional stimulation and the encouragement for this book have come in large part from two academic departments. The faculty of the Department of Epidemiology, Johns Hopkins School of Hygiene and Public Health, taught me the intellectual framework and provided guidance in pursuing epidemiological ideas. The Department of Health Care Sciences at The George Washington University School of Medicine and Health Sciences, with the encouragement of Dr. John Ott, Department Chairman, provided the opportunities to put these ideas into practice. The students, residents, and faculty of the department have provided invaluable feedback.

Melanie Gehen-Benedict, June Blaszkicwicz, and Ed Rovera deserve special thanks for putting together the manuscript and for contending with the revisions of the revisions. I especially thank my wife, Linda, who put herself and her enthusiasm into this project and patiently and skillfully reviewed every word.

Much of the material in Chapters 3 to 7 has been adapted from articles I wrote that first appeared in *Postgraduate Medicine,* May—September 1979, entitled "Interpreting Medical Studies: A Series."

Contents

Studying a Study PART I

Introduction and Sample Test

The traditional course in reading the medical literature consists of "Here's the *New England Journal of Medicine*. Read it!" This approach is analogous to learning to swim by the total immersion method. Some people can learn to swim this way, of course, but a few drown and many learn to fear the water. Reading only the abstracts of medical articles is much like fearing the water.

In contrast to the method of total immersion, what will be presented here is a step-by-step, active-participation approach to a clinical review of the medical literature. With these analytical techniques, the clinician should be able to read a journal article critically and efficiently. There will be considerable emphasis on the errors that can occur in the various kinds of studies, but try to remember that every flaw is not fatal.

Before developing and illustrating the elements of critical analysis, however, let's begin with a flaw-catching exercise, a simulated journal article, and see how well you can do. Read the following study and then try to answer the accompanying questions.

A Prospective Study of Medical Screening in a Military Population

During their first year in the military service, 10,000 18-year-old privates were offered the opportunity to participate in a yearly health maintenance examination that included history, physical examination, and multiple laboratory tests. The first year 5,000 participated and 5,000 failed to participate; the 5,000 participants were selected as a study group, and the 5,000 nonparticipants were selected as a control group. The first-year participants were then offered yearly health maintenance examinations during each year of their military service.

Upon discharge from the military, each of the 5,000 study group members and each of the 5,000 control group members were given an extensive history, physical examination, and laboratory evaluation to determine whether the yearly health maintenance visits had made any difference in health and life style of the participants.

The investigators obtained the following information:

1. On the basis of their reported consumption, participants had half the rate of alcoholism as nonparticipants.

2. Participants had twice as many diagnoses made for them during military service as nonparticipants.
3. Participants had advanced an average of twice as many ranks as nonparticipants.
4. There were no statistically significant differences between the groups in the rate of myocardial infarction.
5. There were no differences between the groups in the rate of development of testicular cancer or Hodgkin's disease, the two most common cancers in young men.

The authors then drew the following conclusions:

1. Yearly screening can reduce the rate of alcoholism in the military by one-half.
2. Since participants had twice the number of diagnoses made for them, their diseases were being diagnosed at an earlier stage in the disease process, at a point where therapy is more beneficial.
3. Since participants had twice the military advancement of nonparticipants, the screening program must have contributed to the quality of their work.
4. Since there was no difference in the rate of myocardial infarction, screening and intervention for coronary risk factors should not be included in a future health maintenance screening program.
5. Since testicular cancer and Hodgkin's disease occurred with equal frequency in both groups, future health maintenance examinations should not include efforts to diagnose these conditions.

Now see if you can answer the following questions, which form the uniform framework for reviewing medical studies.

1. Was the study properly designed to answer the study questions?
2. Was the method of assignment of patients to study and control groups proper?
3. Was the assessment of the results in the study group and in the control group adequately performed?
4. Did the analysis properly compare the outcome in the study and the control groups?

5. Was a valid interpretation drawn from the comparisons made between the study and control groups?
6. Were the extrapolations to individuals not involved in the study properly performed?

How did you do? If you feel you can answer these questions already, turn to the critique on page 87 and compare your answers. If and when you are ready, let's proceed!

Let us begin by outlining a uniform framework for analyzing clinical research articles. It will constitute the foundation for the entire process of studying a study.

The uniform framework contains the following basic components:

ASSIGNMENT   Selection of individuals for a study and a control group

ASSESSMENT   Determination of the results of the investigation in the study and the control groups

ANALYSIS   Comparison of the results of the study and control groups

INTERPRETATION   Drawing conclusions about the meaning of any differences found between the study and control groups

EXTRAPOLATION   Drawing conclusions about the meaning of the study for individuals not included in the study

Figure 2-1 outlines the application of the uniform framework to a research study.

Three basic types of clinical research studies are frequently found in the medical literature: retrospective or case-control studies, prospective or cohort studies, and experimental studies or clinical trials. The uniform framework can be applied to all three types of studies with only minor modifications.

In order to illustrate the application of the uniform framework to retrospective, prospective, and experimental studies, the essential features of each type of study are outlined and then applied to the specific problem of the relationship between estrogen use and uterine cancer.

Retrospective Study
(Case-control Study)

The unique feature of retrospective studies is that they begin after individuals already have developed or failed to develop the disease being investigated. They go back in time to determine the characteristics of individuals prior to the onset of disease. Retrospective studies also are called *case-control studies,* the "cases" being the individuals who have developed the disease already, and the controls

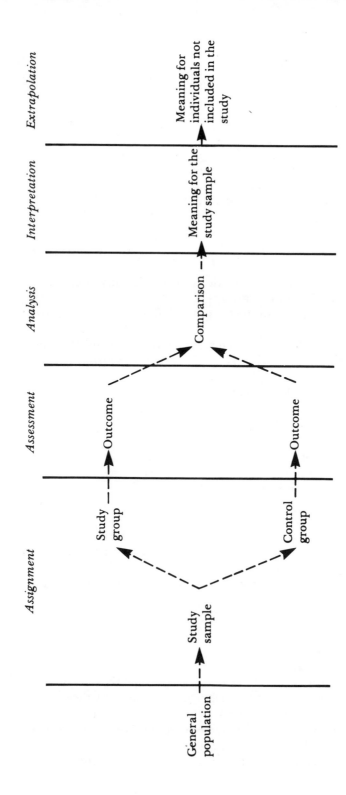

FIGURE 2-1. Uniform framework for studying a study.

being the individuals who have not developed the disease. In order to use a retrospective study to examine the relationship between estrogen use and uterine cancer, an investigator would proceed as follows.

ASSIGNMENT. Select a group of women who currently have uterine cancer (cases) and a group of otherwise similar women who do not have uterine cancer (controls). Since the development of the disease is observed to occur without the investigator's intervention, this process will be called observed assignment.

ASSESSMENT. Determine whether each woman previously took estrogens and, if so, how much she used.

ANALYSIS. Calculate the probability that the group of women with uterine cancer had been estrogen users versus the probability that the group of women without cancer had been estrogen users.

INTERPRETATION. Draw conclusions about the meaning of the differences in the probability of estrogen use by the uterine cancer study group as opposed to the control group.

EXTRAPOLATION. Draw conclusions about the meaning of estrogen use for other women not included in the study.

Figure 2-2 illustrates the application of the uniform framework to this study.

Prospective Study
(Cohort Study)

The unique feature of prospective studies is that they begin *before* individuals have developed the disease that is being investigated and follow them forward in time to determine who subsequently will develop the disease. Prospective studies also are called *cohort studies,* a cohort being a group of individuals who share a common experience. Prospective or cohort studies follow a cohort that possesses the characteristic under study as well as a cohort that does not possess that particular characteristic. In order to use a prospective study to examine the relationship between estrogen use and uterine cancer, an investigator would proceed as follows.

ASSIGNMENT. Select a study group of women who are using estrogens and an otherwise similar control group of women who are not and have not been using estrogens. Since the use of estrogens is observed to occur without the investigator's intervention, this process also will be called observed assignment.

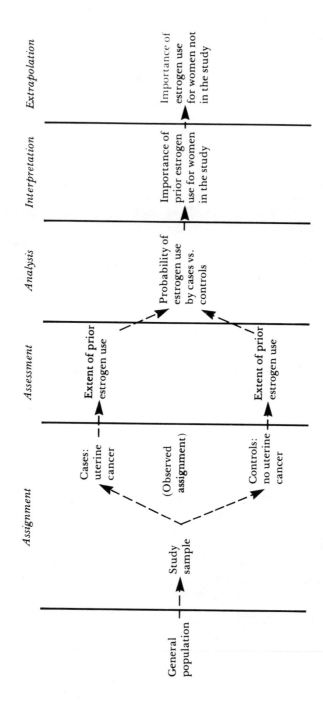

FIGURE 2-2. Application of the uniform framework to a retrospective or case-control study.

ASSESSMENT. Follow these women to determine who subsequently develops uterine cancer.

ANALYSIS. Calculate the risk of developing uterine cancer for women using estrogens versus women not using estrogens.

INTERPRETATION. Draw conclusions about the meaning of the differences in the risk of developing uterine cancer in the study group as opposed to the control group.

EXTRAPOLATION. Draw conclusions about the meaning of these cancer risks for women not included in the study.

Figure 2-3 illustrates the prospective or cohort study.

Experimental Study
(Clinical Trial)

Experimental clinical studies are also called clinical trials. Like prospective studies, individuals are followed forward in time to determine if they develop a particular disease or condition under investigation. The unique feature of experimental studies, however, is the method for assigning individuals to groups. In an experimental study individuals are assigned randomly and blindly either to a study group or to a control group. *Random assignment* means that any one individual has an equal probability of being assigned to the study or the control group. *Blind assignment*—also called *double-blind assignment*—means that neither the participants nor the investigators know whether the participants have been assigned to the study or to the control group. In order to use an experimental study to examine the relationship between estrogens and uterine cancer, an investigator would proceed as follows.

ASSIGNMENT. Blindly and randomly assign women to a study group that will be given estrogen and to a nonestrogen-taking control group.

ASSESSMENT. Follow these women to determine who subsequently develops uterine cancer.

ANALYSIS. Calculate the probability of developing uterine cancer for women using estrogen versus women not using estrogen.

INTERPRETATION. Draw conclusions about the meaning of the differences in the probability of developing uterine cancer in the study group as opposed to the control group.

EXTRAPOLATION. Draw conclusions about the meaning of the difference for women not included in the study.

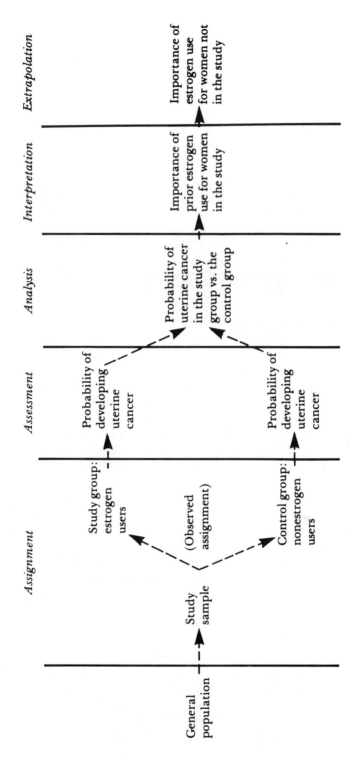

FIGURE 2-3. Application of the uniform framework to a prospective or cohort study.

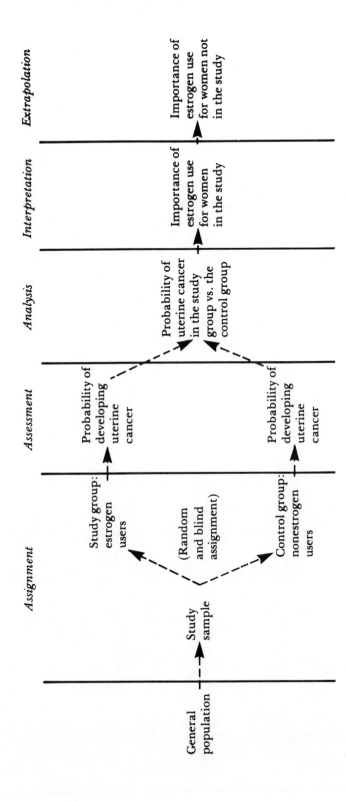

FIGURE 2-4. Application of the uniform framework to an experimental study.

Following the same format as the retrospective and prospective study, Figure 2-4 illustrates the experimental study or clinical trial.

This brief presentation of the three basic study types used in clinical studies is designed merely to show how each type of study can be analyzed by using the uniform framework. In the chapter on study design, the strength and weakness of each study type will be discussed. Before proceeding further with study design, however, let us discuss the requirements for proper implementation of each element of the uniform framework and illustrate the common errors that can occur.

The assignment of individuals to study and control groups is the first component of the uniform framework. In all types of studies investigators attempt to produce study and control groups that are identical in all respects except for the characteristic under study.

Retrospective and prospective studies are called observational studies because the investigators merely observe the assignment of individuals to study and control groups. Moreover, in retrospective studies investigators can observe only that individuals have or do not have a disease, and in prospective studies they can observe only that individuals have or do not have a particular study characteristic. These restrictions are limitations in retrospective and prospective studies that can lead to the error known as selection bias.

Selection Bias

Few terms used in medicine are less clearly understood or more loosely used than the word *bias*. *Webster's New World Dictionary* defines *bias* as "prejudice, a judgment or opinion formed before the fact." According to the best tradition of scientific research, a study should be free of prejudice. Yet, even with the best of scientific intentions, investigators can unintentionally introduce factors into the selection of the study population that predetermine the outcome of the study. These factors are known as selection bias. The elements of selection bias are illustrated in the following hypothetical study.*

An investigation was conducted to compare the contraceptive failure rate of intrauterine devices (IUDs) versus that of birth control pills. Previous studies have shown that the greatest single factor in IUD failure is the high rate of early expulsion while most oral contraceptive failures occur when women do not take the pills as prescribed. The authors selected 10,000 consecutive women with IUDs in place for at least 1 year, and 10,000 consecutive pill users. They found a contraceptive failure rate of 8 per 100 among pill users and 5 per 100 among IUD users. The difference was statistically significant. The authors concluded that the IUD has a lower failure rate than birth control pills.

*In reviewing this hypothetical case as well as the others in the book, the reader should assume that all omitted portions of the study were properly performed.

In light of previous studies, the conclusion that the IUD has a lower failure rate than do birth control pills is a surprising and probably erroneous conclusion. A possible reason for these results is the presence of selection bias. Let us look at how selection bias could have crept into this study. The first question to ask is whether the IUD users chosen for this study were representative of all IUD users. As indicated, each of the women chosen had an IUD in place; therefore they were IUD retainers. The women who had experienced early explusion and did not have the IUD reinserted were IUD users at one time. However, they were not included in the study population since they did not have an IUD in place at the time of the study. Thus, the study population of IUD users was not representative of all IUD users.

The second question one must ask is whether this uniqueness or lack of representativeness could affect the results of the study. Since early expulsion is believed to be the largest factor in IUD failure, the selection of women who did not experience early expulsion produced a study group with a high likelihood of success. The uniqueness of the study group could have affected the results of the study.

This example illustrates the important features of selection bias: (1) The study population was not representative of all individuals who could have been included, and (2) the factor making these women different could have affected the results.

It is not enough to say only that the study group was different or unrepresentative; this, in and of itself, does not constitute selection bias. In fact, most medical studies are done on populations that are not representative of all individuals who could have been included. Whenever an investigator uses a hospital population or a selected community, the study subjects actually chosen are likely to be different from the total population of individuals who could have been chosen. The failure of those chosen to be representative may affect the ability to generalize the results of the study, but it does not constitute selection bias. For selection bias to be operating, the study population must be different in a way that is likely to affect the results.

The IUD example illustrates selection bias in assignment of patients to a study group. Selection bias can operate also in the assignment of patients to a control population, as in the following hypothetical prospective study.

The effect of cigarette smoking on the development of myocardial infarctions was studied by selecting 10,000 cigarette smokers and 10,000 noncigarette-smoking pipe smokers. Both groups were followed for 10 years. The investigators found that the cigarette smokers had a rate of new myocardial infarction of 4 per 100 while the pipe smokers had a rate of new myocardial infarction of 7 per 100. The results were statistically significant. The investigators concluded that cigarette smokers have a lower risk of myocardial infarctions than noncigarette-smoking pipe smokers.

Despite the statistical significance of this difference, the conclusion is in conflict with the results of many other studies. Let us see if selection bias could have contributed to the results.

In analyzing this study one must recognize the two generally accepted facts that men make up the vast majority of pipe smokers, although both men and women smoke cigarettes, and that men have a much higher rate of myocardial infarction than women.

With these facts in mind, the first question to ask is whether the selection of noncigarette-smoking, pipe smokers as controls was representative of all noncigarette smokers. Obviously not: since men constitute the vast majority of pipe smokers, the individuals chosen as controls were not representative of all noncigarette smokers in that the control group included a much higher proportion of men.

The second question to ask is whether it is likely that the uniqueness of the control group affected the results. The answer is yes: men have a higher risk of myocardial infarction and men were disproportionately represented among the noncigarette smokers. Thus, one would expect the heavily male control group to have a higher myocardial infarction rate regardless of the effect of pipe smoking. This study, then, incorporates both elements of selection bias. The control subjects were different enough from those who could have been selected so that the outcome was affected.

These examples illustrate selection bias in the assignment of individuals to both the study group and the control group in a prospective study. Retrospective studies may also suffer from selection bias as is shown in the following example.

A retrospective study of the causes of premenopausal breast cancer compared the past use of birth control pills among 500 females with breast cancer to the past use of the pills among 500 age-matched women admitted for hypertension or diabetes. They found that 40% of the women with breast cancer had used birth control pills during the preceeding five years while only 5% of those with diabetes or hypertension in the control group had used the pills. The authors concluded that there was a strong association between the use of birth control pills and the development of premenopausal breast cancer.

In order to determine whether a selection bias existed in the assignment of patients to the control group, one must first ask whether the patients were representative of women without breast cancer. The answer is no, since these women were unique in being admitted to the hospital for diabetes or hypertension. One must then ask whether their uniqueness was likely to have affected the probability of their use of the characteristic under study, that is, birth control pills. The answer is yes: since birth control pills are widely known to increase blood pressure and blood sugar, physicians are not likely to prescribe birth control pills to women with hypertension and diabetes. Thus the uniqueness of the health of these women contributed to a lower-than-expected use of birth control pills. This study therefore incorporated a selection bias in the assignment of patients.

Comparability

In both retrospective and prospective studies, proper study design can often eliminate selection bias. In experimental studies, selection bias is avoided by randomly and blindly assigning individuals to study and control groups. Careful study design of retrospective, prospective, or even experimental studies, however, does not assure that the study and control groups will actually be similar. Chance alone may result in important differences between the groups in all three types of studies.

To determine whether chance differences have occurred, the investigators should attempt to define a broad range of potentially relevant characteristics of the study group and of the control group. They then should compare the two groups to determine whether they are in fact similar. This is especially important for any factors that might be related to outcome. Chance alone, even with proper study design, may produce differences between groups that place one group at greater risk of developing the condition under study.

Thus, even though no selection bias has occurred and blind,

random assignment has been performed, the groups may differ by chance in a factor related to outcome. The consequences of this lack of comparability, even in an experimental study, is illustrated in the following hypothetical study.

To evaluate the effectiveness of a new medication for coronary artery disease, an experimental trial was conducted. One hundred patients were randomly and blindly assigned to a treatment group and 100 patients to a placebo group. The treatment group had an average age of 58, while the placebo control group had an average age of 65. The authors found that during the next five years the control group experienced twice the rate of myocardial infarction. The authors argued that since they had randomly and blindly assigned patients to both the treatment and placebo groups, the differences in age of the two groups was of no consequence.

Even with random and blind allocation from the same patient population as ideally performed in a controlled clinical trial, there may by chance be important differences between the control and study groups. Despite the fact that differences in age were the result of chance, age is certainly related to the probability of developing coronary artery disease. Thus age differences between the study and control groups indicate that the groups differ in a factor that affects their risk of developing the condition under study. A factor such as age, which differs between the study and control groups and is likely to affect outcome, is known as a *confounding variable* (See Chap. 5).

The existence of a confounding variable does not invalidate an investigation. If the lack of comparable groups is recognized, the differences can be taken into account in the analysis. It is important therefore to recognize those differences between the study group and the control group that can affect the outcome of a study.

Assessment of
Outcome

Having examined the process of assignment of individuals to study and control groups, let us turn our attention to the second component of the uniform framework, the assessment of results. To assess the results of a study, the researchers must define an outcome that they intend to measure. The term *outcome* can be somewhat confusing because it has different meanings for the different types of studies. Let us review what outcome means in each of our basic study types and then define the criteria for a valid measure of outcome.

Both prospective and experimental studies begin with a study group that possesses the characteristic under study and a control group that is free of this characteristic. Individuals in the study group are followed forward in time to determine whether they will develop a particular condition. In both studies, the condition that is hypothesized is known as the outcome. The investigator must employ a valid measure of the presence of the condition. For instance, in the estrogen use and uterine cancer examples (pp. 9, 11), the development of uterine cancer is the outcome assessed by investigators.

Retrospective studies begin with persons who have already developed a certain condition (cases) and persons who have not developed the condition (controls). The investigators review the past history of individuals in both the case and the control groups to determine whether these individuals had exposure to, or possession of, a hypothesized prior characteristic. In a restrospective study this prior characteristic is the outcome or result of the study. A valid measure of the outcome or prior characteristic must be employed by investigators. In the estrogen use and uterine cancer example given previously (p. 9) the use of estrogens is the outcome being assessed.

What constitutes a valid measure of outcome? Each of the following criteria must be satisfied.

1. The investigator must use a measure of outcome that is *appropriate* to the question to be answered.
2. The measurement of outcome must be *precise*.
3. The measurement of outcome must be *complete*.
4. The outcome of the study must not be influenced by the *process of observation*.

Appropriate Measure of Outcome

To understand the importance of the appropriateness of a measure of outcome, let us first consider an example of how the use of an inappropriate measure of outcome can invalidate a study's conclusions.

An investigator attempts to study the relationship between urban living conditions and later development of active tuberculosis (TB) in a country with a high rate of active TB. Five hundred infants from a poor urban area are compared with 500 infants from a poor rural area. The investigator follows the children for 10 years and finds that 70% of the urban children develop a positive TB skin test versus 10% of the rural children. The investigator concludes that urban living is associated with the development of active TB.

A TB skin test does not evaluate the *presence* of active TB; it assesses previous *exposure*. Thus the investigator has not measured what he thought he had measured. The experiment may have established evidence for greater exposure of children to TB in urban areas, but since the intent was to measure the development of active TB, an inappropriate—and invalid—measure of outcome was used. The conclusion reached is therefore not valid either.

Precise Measure of Outcome

Next we will look at how an outcome may be affected by imprecise measurements. Information for measuring outcome may come from three sources:

1. Reports by study individuals
2. Readings from testing instruments
3. Measurements by the study investigator

Any of these sources may produce imprecise data.

REPORTS BY STUDY INDIVIDUALS

Information from study individuals is subject to recall and reporting errors. *Recall errors* imply defects in memory, especially defects in which one group is more likely to recall events than the other group. *Reporting errors* occur when one group of study subjects is more accurate than the other in reporting what they remember. Consider the following example of how recall errors can occur.

In a retrospective study of the cause of spina bifida, 100 mothers of infants born with the disease and 100 mothers of infants born without the disease are studied. Of the mothers of spina bifida infants 50% report having had a sore throat during pregnancy versus 5% of the mothers whose infants did not develop spina bifida. The investigators conclude that they have shown an association between sore throats during pregnancy and spina bifida.

Before accepting the conclusion of the study, one must ask whether recall error could explain its findings. One can argue that mothers who experienced the trauma of having an infant with spina bifida are likely to search their memory more intensely and to remember events not usually recalled by other women. That is, recall bias is more likely to occur when the subsequent events are traumatic, causing inconsequential prior events to be recalled that under normal circumstances are usually forgotten. Thus, the result of the study may be attributable, at least in part, to recall error, and doubt is cast on the alleged association between sore throats during pregnancy and occurrence of spina bifida.

Reporting error (as well as recall error) may operate to impair the precision, and therefore the validity, of assessment as illustrated in the following example.

A study of the relationship between gonorrhea and multiple sexual partners was conducted. One hundred women newly diagnosed as having gonorrhea were compared with 100 women in the same clinical population found to be free of gonorrhea. The women diagnosed as having gonorrhea were informed that the serious consequences of the disease could be prevented only by locating and treating sexual partners. Both groups of women were asked about the number of sexual partners they had during the preceding two months. The gonorrhea group reported an average of twice as many sexual partners. The investigators concluded that women with gonorrhea have twice as many sexual partners as women without gonorrhea.

It can be argued that the women with gonorrhea in this study felt a greater obligation, hence less hesitation, to report their sexual partners than did the women without the disease. Reporting errors are more likely to occur when the nature of the information sought is confidential and/or when one group is under more pressure than another group to report previous events accurately. In short, reporting error along with recall error may operate to impair the precision of assessment. Thus, the women with gonorrhea may simply have been more thorough in reporting their sexual partners rather than actually having more contacts.

INSTRUMENT ERROR

Error in measurement may also occur with imprecise measurement by the testing instruments, as illustrated in the following example.

The side effects of a new anti-inflammatory drug were evaluated by blindly and randomly selecting half the members of a rheumatoid arthritis study population to receive the new drug and half to receive placebos. To evaluate the risk of gastritis, the investigators put all patients through an upper GI series at the end of the course of medication. The investigators found no evidence that the new drug causes gastritis.

The investigators did not recognize that an upper GI series is a very poor instrument for measuring gastritis. Even if the new drug causes gastritis, upper GI X-ray examination would not be adequate to identify its presence. Thus any conclusion based on this measurement is invalid. When gross instrument error occurs, as in this example, the measurement of outcome also can be considered inappropriate.

INVESTIGATOR ERROR

Whenever the measurement of outcome depends on subjective interpretation of data, the possibility of misinterpretation always exists. Even properly designed studies cannot entirely eliminate these errors. It is possible, however, to recognize and correct for a fundamental principle of human psychology, namely, that people, including investigators, see what they want to see or expect to see. This is accomplished by keeping the investigator—who makes the assessment of outcome—from knowing an individual's group assignment. Blind assessment can be utilized in retrospective and prospective studies as well as experimental studies. Failure to use blind assessment can lead to the following type of error.

In the previous study, the investigators, who assigned individuals to drug and placebo groups, tried to determine whether the drug group patients had more symptoms compatible with gastritis than did the patients in the placebo group. After questioning all patients about their symptoms, they determined that there was no increase in the incidence of gastritis caused by the drug. They reported that the data conformed with their hypothesis that the new drug did not cause gastritis.

In this study the investigators making the assessment of outcome were aware of which patients were receiving the drug and which were receiving the placebo; they were not "blinded." In addition, they were assessing the patient's subjective symptoms such as nausea and stomach pain or indigestion in deciding whether gastritis was present. Since the assessment conformed with their own hypothesis, their results are open to question. This does not imply fraud, only the natural tendency of human beings to see what they expect or want to see. The investigators' conclusions *may be* valid, but their less than perfect techniques make it difficult or impossible to accept their conclusion.

Completeness of Assessment

Whenever follow-up of patients is incomplete, the possibility exists that those not included in the final assessment had a different outcome from those included. The following example illustrates an error due to incomplete assessment.

In a study of the effect of a new alcohol treatment program, 100 patients are assigned to a new alcohol treatment program and 100 patients are given conventional treatment. The investigator visits the homes of all the patients at 9:00 on a Saturday night and draws blood from all available patients for measuring alcohol level. Of the new treatment group, 30 patients were at home and one-third of these had alcohol in their blood. Among the conventionally treated patients, 40 were at home and one-half of these had alcohol in their blood. The authors conclude that the new treatment reduced subsequent drinking more than did the conventional treatment.

It can be argued that in this study, a number of those who could not be located were not available because they were out drinking. If this were the case, the results of the study might have been dramatically altered with complete follow-up. Incomplete follow-up can invalidate the conclusions of an investigation.

Incomplete follow-up does not necessarily mean that the patients are lost to follow-up as in the previous example. They may be followed to varying extents as the following example illustrates.

A study of the side effects of birth control pills was conducted by comparing 1,000 young women on the pill with 1,000 young women on other forms of birth control. Data were collected from the records of their private physicians over a one-year period. Pill users were scheduled for three follow-up visits during the year; other women were asked to return if they had problems. Among users of the pill, 75 reported having headaches, 90 reported fatigue, and 60 reported depression. Among nonpill users, 25 patients reported having headaches, 30 reported fatigue, and 20 reported depression. The average pill user made three visits to her physician during the year versus one visit for the nonpill user. The investigators concluded that use of the pill is associated with increased frequency of headaches, fatigue, and depression.

The problem of unequal observation of the two groups may have invalidated the results. The fact that pill users made three times as many visits to the physician may account for the more frequent recordings of headache, fatigue, and depression. With more frequent observation, frequently occurring subjective symptoms are more likely to be reported.

Effect of Observation

Even if a study meets the difficult criteria of appropriate, precise, and complete assessment, there is one more threat to its validity. Investigators intend to measure events as they would have occurred had no one been watching. Unfortunately, the very process of conducting a study involves the introduction of an observer into the events being measured. Thus, the reviewer must determine whether the process of observation altered the outcome. An example follows in which this may have occurred.

A study was conducted of the relationship between smoking and coronary artery disease. One thousand male smokers, age 50, and 1,000 male nonsmokers, age 50, were followed for 10 years to evaluate the effects of smoking on coronary artery disease. Other risk factors were equally distributed between the groups. At the end of 10 years there was no difference in the rate of coronary artery disease. The authors also found that 60% of the smokers had stopped smoking during the 10-year study period. The authors concluded that this study helped refute any relationship between smoking and coronary artery disease.

Whenever it is possible for study subjects to switch groups or alter their behavior, the effects of observation may invalidate an investigation. This is most likely to occur when the study subjects also are aware of the possibility that their behavior may harm their health. The additional element of observation may have tipped the scales, causing smokers to do what they knew they should do anyway.

Having discussed assignment and assessment, let us proceed to the third component of the uniform framework: analysis of the results. As the investigators compare results in both the study and control groups, they try to adjust for, or to take into account, factors other than those being studied that may account for the results. After making these adjustments, the investigators usually will perform a statistical significance test.

Adjustment

It was pointed out in Chapter 3 that the investigator is obliged to compare the individual characteristics of the study group with those of the control group to determine whether they differ in any way. If the groups differ, the investigator must consider whether these differences could have affected the results. Differences between groups that may affect the results of the study are potential *confounding variables.* These confounding variables may result either from selection bias in retrospective or prospective studies or from chance differences in all three types of studies. If a potential confounding variable is detected, the investigator is obliged to take this into consideration in the analysis with a process known as adjustment of data.

In performing an adjustment, the investigator separates into groups those who possess different levels of the confounding variable. Groups with the same level of confounding variable are then compared to see if the differences persist. For instance, if age is a potential confounding variable, the investigator subdivides the groups by age into several categories; then the study and control groups in each age classification are compared to determine whether differences persist when the effects of age are eliminated. Sophisticated statistical techniques known as multiple regression are available for adjusting more than one factor at a time (see Part 4, *Selecting a Statistic*). Failure to recognize and adjust for a confounding variable can result in serious errors as illustrated in the following example.

An investigator studied the relationship between coffee consumption and lung cancer by following 500 heavy coffee drinkers and 500 noncoffee drinkers for 10 years. In this prospective study, the risk of lung cancer in heavy coffee drinkers was 10 times that of coffee abstainers. The author concluded that coffee, along with cigarettes, was established as a risk factor in the development of lung cancer.

Cigarette smoking may be considered a confounding variable in this study if it is assumed that cigarette smoking is associated with coffee drinking; in other words, coffee drinkers are more likely than noncoffee drinkers to smoke cigarettes. Furthermore, cigarettes are associated with lung cancer. Thus, cigarettes are a potential confounding factor related both to the study characteristic of coffee drinking, and to the outcome of lung cancer. If cigarette smoking is a confounding variable, adjustment for cigarette smoking must be performed as part of the analysis.

In adjusting for cigarette smoking, the investigation would divide coffee drinkers into cigarette smokers and noncigarette smokers, and would do the same with the noncoffee drinkers. The investigator would then compare nonsmoking, coffee drinkers with nonsmoking, noncoffee drinkers to determine if the relationship between coffee drinking and lung cancer still holds true. Only after determining that adjustment for cigarette smoking does not eliminate the relationship between coffee drinking and lung cancer can the author conclude that coffee drinking is associated with the development of lung cancer.

Prior Matching

Another method for circumventing the problem of confounding variables is to match individuals prior to the study. Investigators would choose individuals for both the study and control groups who are similar with respect to a confounding variable. For instance, if age is related to the probability of getting into either group, and if age is also related to outcome, then the investigators may match for age. For every 65-year-old in the control group, investigators would choose one 65-year-old for the study group, and similarly with 30-year-olds, 40-year-olds, and so on. If properly performed, the result of matching is a guarantee that the average age of each group will be similar.

Matching is not limited to making the groups uniform for age. It may be used for any factor that is a confounding variable, that is, for a factor related both to the probability of being included in the assigned group and to the probability of experiencing the outcome. For example, if one were studying the relationship between birth control pills and strokes, then blood pressure would be considered a confounding variable. Since high blood pressure is a relative contraindication to the use of birth control pills, high blood pressure would lower the probability of a person's being assigned to the birth control pill group. In addition, since high blood pressure also is known to increase the probability of strokes, high blood pressure also would affect the probability of developing the outcome. Therefore, blood pressure is a confounding variable on which one might want to match the groups.

One disadvantage of matching groups is that the investigators cannot study the effects of the factor on which they matched the groups. For instance, if they match for age and blood pressure, they lose the ability to study the effect of age and blood pressure on the development of strokes. Furthermore, they lose the ability to study factors which are closely associated with the matched factor. The pitfall in attempting to study the matched factor or closely linked factors is illustrated in the following example.

One hundred adult-onset diabetics were compared to 100 nondiabetic adults who were matched for relative weight in order to study factors associated with adult-onset diabetes. The authors found that the total calories consumed in each of the two groups was nearly identical and concluded that the number of calories consumed was not related to the possibility of developing adult-onset diabetes.

The authors of the study, having matched the patients by weight, then attempted to study the differences in calories consumed. Since there is a high level of correlation between weight and calories consumed, it is not surprising that the authors found no difference in consumption of calories between the two groups matched for weight. In general it is not possible to study matching factors or factors closely associated with the matched factors.

Statistical Significance Testing
Most investigations are conducted on only a sample or segment of the larger group of individuals who could have been included in the study. Researchers therefore are frequently confronted with the question of whether they would achieve similar results if the larger population were used or whether chance selection has pro-

duced unusual results in their study. Unfortunately, there is no direct method for answering this question; instead, investigators are forced to test their study hypothesis using a circuitous method of proof by elimination. This method is known as statistical significance testing.

Statistical significance testing is a probability method that attempts to quantitate from the study data the likelihood of obtaining the observed data if no true difference between groups or association between factors actually exists in the larger population.

In strict statistical terms, statistical significance testing assumes that the study group and the control group are representative of all those who could have been included in the study. Both the study and the control groups should be random samples of all those who could have been included. This use of the term *random* is confusing because statistical significance testing does not require that the assignment of individuals to a study or a control group be randomly performed as is done in an experimental study. Random selection is required, randomization is not.

SIGNIFICANCE TESTING PROCEDURES

Statistical significance testing begins with a study hypothesis stating that a difference between groups or an association of factors exists in the larger population. In performing statistical significance tests, it is assumed initially that the study hypothesis is false, and a null hypothesis is formulated stating that no difference or association exists in the larger population. Statistical methods then are used to calculate the probability of obtaining the observed results in the study sample if the null hypothesis were true. In other words, statistical significance tests measure the probability of obtaining the observed study results if no true difference or association actually exists in the larger population.

When only a small probability exists that the observed results would occur if the null hypothesis were true, then investigators can reject the null hypothesis. In rejecting the null hypothesis, the investigators accept by elimination the existence of a difference or association in the larger population. The specific steps in statistical significance testing proceed as follows.

1. State hypothesis: Before collecting the data, the investigators state a study hypothesis that a difference exists between the study group and the control group.

2. Formulate null hypothesis: The investigators then assume that no true difference exists between the study group and the control group. This is known as the "null" hypothesis.

3. Decide significance level: The investigators determine what level of probability or significance will be considered small enough to reject the null hypothesis. In a majority of clinical studies, a 5% chance or less of occurrence is considered unlikely enough to allow the investigator to reject the null hypothesis. The 5% figure, although traditional, is clinically arbitrary. It leaves open the possibility that chance alone has produced an unusual set of data. Thus a null hypothesis, which is in fact true, could be rejected in favor of the study hypothesis.

4. Collect data: The data may be collected using a retrospective, prospective or experimental study.

5. Apply statistical significance test: If differences between the sample groups exist, the investigators attempt to quantitate the probability that these differences would occur if no true differences exist between the larger populations from which both the study and control group individuals have been selected. In other words, they calculate the probability that the observed data would occur if the null hypothesis of no difference were true. In order to do so, the investigators must choose from among a variety of statistical significance tests, each one of which is appropriate to a different type of data. Therefore, investigators must be careful that they have chosen the proper test. (See Part 4, *Selecting a Statistic*.)

To understand how a statistical significance test measures probability, let us look at an example that uses numbers small enough to allow for easy calculation. Assume that an investigator wants to study the question, "Are there an equal number of males and females born in the United States?" The investigator first hypothesizes that more males than females are born in the U.S.; he then formulates a null hypothesis that an equal number of males and females are born in the U.S. Next, he samples four birth certificates and finds that there are four males and zero females in his sample of births. Let us now calculate the probability of obtaining four males and zero females if the null hypothesis of equal numbers of males and females is true.

Probability of one male	50%
Probability of two males in a row	25%
Probability of three males in a row	12½%
Probability of four males in a row	6¼%

Thus there is a 6¼% chance of obtaining four males in a row even if there are an equal number of males and females born in the United States. A simple form of significance test such as this one can yield the probability of producing the observed data assuming that the null hypothesis is true. All statistical significance tests yield similar types of results. They all measure the probability of obtaining the observed data if no true differences between groups actually exist in the larger population.

6. Reject or fail to reject the null hypothesis: Having determined the probability that the results could have occurred by chance if no true difference exists in the larger population, the investigators proceed to reject or fail to reject the null hypothesis. If the probability of the results occurring by chance is less than or equal to 5%, investigators can reject the null hypothesis thereby indicating that the probability is very small that chance alone could explain the differences in outcome. By elimination they accept the proposition that there is a true difference in the outcome between the larger population of study individuals and the larger population of control individuals from which the research individuals were selected.

What if the probability of occurrence by chance is greater than 5% as in the preceding example? The investigators then are unable to reject the null hypothesis, which does not mean that the null hypothesis of no true difference in the larger population is true. It merely indicates that the probability of obtaining the observed results, if the null hypothesis were true, is too great to reject the null hypothesis in favor of the study hypothesis. The burden of proof, therefore, is on the investigators to show that the null hypothesis is quite unlikely before rejecting it in favor of the study hypothesis. The following example shows how the significance testing procedure operates in practice.

An investigator wanted to test the hypothesis that mouth cancer is associated with pipe smoking. She formulated a null hypothesis stating that pipe smoking is not associated with mouth cancer in the general population. She then decided that if she obtained data that would occur only 5% or less of the time if the null hypothesis were true, she would reject the null hypothesis. She next collected data from a sample of the general population of pipe smokers and nonpipe smokers. Using the proper statistical significance test, she found that if there were no association between pipe smoking and mouth cancer then her data would have occurred by chance alone only 3% of the time. She now concluded that since her data was quite unlikely to occur if there was no association between pipe smoking and mouth cancer in the general population, she would reject the null hypothesis. The investigator thus accepted by elimination the study hypothesis that there is an association between pipe smoking and mouth cancer in the general population.

Remember that we have defined *small* as a 5% probability or less that the observed results would have occurred if no true difference exists in the larger population. The 5% figure may be too large if important decisions rest on the results. The 5% figure is based on some convenient statistical properties; however, for medical purposes it is completely arbitrary. It is possible to define *small* as 1%, 0.1%, or as any other probability one chooses. Remember, however, that no matter what level is chosen, there will always be some probability of rejecting the null hypothesis when no true difference exists. Statistical significance tests can measure this probability but they cannot eliminate it.

P VALUES

The results of statistical significance tests are usually presented as "p" values. A p value or level of statistical significance indicates the probability of obtaining the observed differences or association in the sample data if there is no true difference or association in the larger parent population. A p value of .05, for instance, indicates a 5% probability of achieving the observed difference or association if the null hypothesis of no true difference or association is true. Similarly a p value of .001 means that there is 1 chance in 1,000 of obtaining the observed difference or association if the null hypothesis is true. Table 5-1 reviews and summarizes the steps in performing a statistical significance test.

Errors in Significance Tests

There are several types of errors that commonly occur in utilizing statistical significance tests:

TABLE 5-1. HOW A STATISTICAL SIGNIFICANCE TEST WORKS

1. *State hypothesis*
   Develop the study question: An association exists between factors or a difference exists between groups in the general population.
2. *Formulate null hypothesis*
   Reverse the hypothesis: No association between factors or difference between groups exists in the general population.
3. *Decide significance level*
   ≦5% unless otherwise indicated
4. *Collect data*
   Determine whether an association between factors or a difference between groups exists in the data collected from samples of the larger population.
5. *Apply statistical significance test*
   Determine the probability of obtaining the observed data if the null hypothesis were true, i.e., choose and apply the correct statistical significance test.
6. *Reject or fail to reject the null hypothesis*
   Reject the null hypothesis and accept by elimination the study hypothesis if the significance level is reached. Fail to reject the null hypothesis if the observed data has more than a 5% probability of occurring by chance if there is no association between factors or difference between groups in the larger population.

1. Failure to state the study hypothesis before conducting the study.
2. Failure to correctly interpret the results of statistical significance tests by not considering the Type I and Type II errors inherent in the method.

Let us begin by observing the consequences of failure to state the hypothesis before conducting the study.

An investigator randomly selected 100 individuals known to have essential hypertension and 100 individuals known to be free of hypertension. He compared them according to a list of 100 variables to determine how the two groups differed. Of the 100 variables studied, two were found to be statistically significant at the .05 level using standard statistical methods: 1) Hypertensives generally have more letters in their last name than nonhypertensives; 2) hypertensives generally are born during the first three and a half days of the week while nonhypertensives are usually born during the last three and a half days of the week. The author concluded that, despite the fact that these differences had not been foreseen, longer names and a birth during the first half of the week are statistically associated with essential hypertension.

This example illustrates the importance of stating the hypothesis beforehand. Whenever a large number of variables are tested, it is likely by chance alone that some of them will be statistically significant using the usual methods of testing. It is not surprising that the investigator found some statistically significant variables. If there is no hypothesis stated beforehand, there can be no null hypothesis to reject. In addition, it is not proper to apply the usual levels of statistical significance unless the hypothesis has been stated before collecting and analyzing the data. If associations are looked for only after collecting the data, much stricter criteria must be applied than the usual 5% probability.

TYPE I ERRORS
There are some errors that are inherent in the method. Fundamental to the concept of statistical significance testing is the possibility that a null hypothesis will be falsely rejected and a study hypothesis will be falsely accepted. This is known as a Type I error. In traditional significance testing, there is as much as a 5% probability of incorrectly accepting a study hypothesis even when no true difference exists in the larger population from which the study samples were obtained. Statistical significance testing does not eliminate uncertainty, it merely quantifies it. Careful readers of studies are therefore able to appreciate the degree of doubt that exists and can decide for themselves whether they are willing to tolerate or act upon that degree of uncertainty.

In some circumstances a 5% probability that no true difference or association exists may be more than one is willing to tolerate. In other circumstances one may tolerate even more than a 5% uncertainty. For instance, before introducing a new method of water purification into a community with a low frequency of waterborne infection, one might not tolerate a 5% probability that the new method would fail to kill disease organisms. On the other hand, in a community where water was a major source of disease transmission, one might tolerate a higher than 5% probability that the new method would fail to thoroughly eliminate water-borne disease, especially if no other method were available. Let us see how failure to appreciate the possibility of a Type I error can lead to misinterpretation of study results.

The author of a medical review article evaluated 20 well-conducted studies that examined the relationship between breast feeding and breast cancer. Nineteen of the studies found no association between breast feeding and breast cancer. One study found an association between breast feeding and increased breast cancer significant at the .05 level. The author of the review article concluded that, since a study existed suggesting that breast feeding is associated an increased risk of breast cancer, breast feeding should be discouraged.

When 20 well-conducted studies are performed to test an association that in fact does not exist, one of the studies may show an association at the .05 level simply by chance. Remember the meaning of statistical significance at the .05 level. It implies that the results have a 5% chance or odds of 1 in 20 of occurring by chance alone if no association exists in the larger population. Thus one study in 20 that shows an association should not be interpreted as evidence *for* an association. It is important to keep in mind the possibility that no association may exist even when statistically significant results have been demonstrated. If the only study showing a relationship had been adopted without further questioning, breast feeding might have been discouraged without producing any cancer-prevention benefits.

TYPE II ERRORS

A Type II error is the reverse of a Type I error. It says that failure to reject the null hypothesis does not necessarily mean that no true difference exists. Remember that the burden of proof in statistical significance testing is on those who say that a true difference exists. The process of significance testing allows one to reject or to not reject a null hypothesis. It does not allow one to prove a null hypothesis. Failure to reject a null hypothesis merely implies that the evidence is not strong enough to reject the assumption that no difference between groups or association between factors exists in the larger population.

There are two factors that may prevent an investigator from demonstrating a statistically significant difference even when one exists. Chance alone may produce an unusual set of data that fail to strongly support a difference even though one actually exists in the larger population. This type of error is parallel to a Type I error, indicating that chance has played a part. A particular study may come up with an unusual outcome that could occur only a small percentage of the time. It does not imply that mistakes were made in design or interpretation of the study; it merely points out that, despite the best efforts and intentions, statistical methods can produce incorrect conclusions. This factor is inherent in statistical concepts since every effort to quantify the probability that you are correct carries with it the probability that you are wrong.

In addition to the constant possibility of unusual data occurring by chance, investigators may stack the odds against themselves by using too few individuals in a study. The smaller the number of individuals included in a study, the more difficult it is to produce data that are strong enough to reject the null hypothesis. The smaller the number of individuals included in a study, the larger the true difference must be before statistically significant results can be demonstrated. Conversely, the larger the number of individuals who are included in a study, the smaller the size of the true difference that can be shown to be statistically significant. At its extreme, this concept holds that any true difference, no matter how small, can be shown to be statistically significant if a large enough number of individuals are used in the study.

This concept is analagous to using a high power microscopic lens to see bacteria. The large numbers increase the resolution of the study. They allow one to see smaller differences. Statistical techniques are available for estimating the probability that a study could establish a statistically significant difference if a true difference actually exists in the larger population. These techniques measure the statistical "power" of the study. In many studies the probability is quite large that one will fail to show a statistically significant difference when a true difference actually exists. There is no arbitrary number that indicates how large a Type II error one should tolerate. Without actually stating it, investigators who use relatively small numbers may be accepting a 20%, 30% or even greater risk that they will fail to demonstrate a statistically significant difference even when a true difference exists in the general population.

One must keep in mind that very large numbers allow one to demonstrate statistically significant differences for very small and even inconsequential differences. Conversely, very small numbers may prevent one from demonstrating statistical significance even when substantial differences are present in the general population. Table 5-2 summarizes and compares Type I and Type II errors.

The following example shows the effect of sample size on the ability to demonstrate differences between groups.

A study of the adverse effects of cigarettes on health was undertaken by following 100 cigarette smokers and 100 nonsmokers for 20 years. During the 20 years, five smokers developed lung cancer while none of the nonsmokers were afflicted. During the same time period, 10 smokers and nine nonsmokers developed myocardial infarction. The results for lung cancer were statistically significant, but the results for myocardial infarction were not. The authors concluded that an association between cigarettes and lung cancer had been supported and an association between cigarette smoking and myocardial infarction had been refuted.

When differences between groups are very large, as they are between smokers and nonsmokers in relation to lung cancer, it may require only a relatively small population to demonstrate statistical significance. When the true differences are smaller, it requires larger numbers to demonstrate a difference. This study cannot be said to refute an association between cigarettes and myocardial infarction. It is very likely that the numbers used were too small to give the study enough "power" to demonstrate an asso-

TABLE 5-2. INHERENT ERRORS OF STATISTICAL SIGNIFICANCE TESTING

	Type I Error	Type II Error
Definition:	Rejection of null hypothesis when no true difference exists in the larger population	Failure to reject null hypothesis when a true difference exists in the larger population
Cause:	Chance	Chance or a too small sample size
Likelihood of occurrence:	Setting of significance level will indicate how large an error will be tolerated (usually 5%)	Statistical techniques can estimate occurrence from the size of the groups (probability of error may be quite large if the numbers are small)

ciation between cigarettes and myocardial infarction even though other studies suggest that an association exists in the general population. A study with limited statistical power to demonstrate a difference also has limited power to refute a difference. No statistically significant difference was found for the relationship between cigarette smoking and myocardial infarction. Therefore there is not enough evidence from this study to reject the null hypothesis that no relationship exists between cigarette smoking and myocardial infarction. Using larger numbers, a statistically significant relationship *may* have been shown.

Having analyzed the study results and concluded that a true difference between groups or a true association between factors exists, the careful reviewer or investigator now wants to know what the results mean for those included in the study. In deciding what the study results mean, both the reviewer and the investigator are interpreting the study; they are applying criteria or information from outside the study itself to draw a conclusion about its meaning.

Interpretation usually has one of two goals: 1) deciding the clinical usefulness or importance of the results obtained, or 2) determining whether a cause and effect relationship has been established. Let us look at how the reader and the investigator should address these questions of clinical importance and cause and effect.

Clinical Importance

Two important questions to consider in determining the clinical importance of a statistically significant difference are: 1) Is the difference large enough to be clinically useful? 2) What is the degree of overlap between the groups?

In answering these questions, the reviewer must remember that one of the limitations of a statistical significance test is the fact that even very small differences are likely to be statistically significant if enough individuals are used in a study. In other words, a very large study has the power to demonstrate statistical significance for very small, even clinically inconsequential differences. Let us look at an example that illustrates the consequences of using large numbers of individuals in a study.

Investigators followed 100,000 middle-aged men for ten years to determine which factors were associated with coronary artery disease. They hypothesized beforehand that uric acid might be a factor in predicting the disease. The investigators found that men who developed coronary artery disease had an average uric acid measure of 7.8 while men who did not develop the disease had an average uric acid measure of 7.7. The difference was statistically significant at the .05 level. The authors concluded that, since a statistically significant difference had been found, the results would be clinically useful.

The differences in the above study are statistically significant, but they are so small that they probably are not important clinically. The large number of men under observation allowed investigators to detect a very small difference between groups. However, the small size of the difference makes it unlikely that uric acid measurements could be clinically useful in predicting who will develop coronary artery disease. The small difference does not allow the clinician to differentiate usefully between those who will develop coronary artery disease and those who will not.

There is another limitation to the concept of statistical significance. Whenever the outcome of a study is expressed as a measurement with a spectrum of possible values, the results are expressed as differences between group averages. Thus many statistically significant differences are saying that the difference between the average values in the two groups is unlikely to result by chance alone. The presence of a statistically significant difference tells us little about how close or how diverse the values are for each group. It is possible for the values of the individuals in each group to be close to the average or to vary widely on either side of the average. The values for individuals in one group may overlap the values for individuals in the other group despite the existence of a statistically significant difference.

In an attempt to avoid the problems that arise from this limitation, research results are frequently presented with a measure of the variability or dispersion within each group. This measure is known as a standard deviation. Assuming that the population chosen is approximately distributed in a bell-shaped or normal (Gaussian) distribution, the standard deviation has a convenient property. About 95% of individual values are found within two standard deviations on either side of the average.

Research results are usually presented as an average plus or minus ($\pm$) one standard deviation. This makes it possible to estimate easily how much overlap there is between two populations. For example, assume that population A has scores of 80 ± 10. The 80 here is the average and 10 is one standard deviation. Assume that population B has scores of 60 ± 15. Remember that 95% of the individuals in each population will have scores within two standard deviations of the average.

For population A with scores of 80 ± 10, two standard deviations equal 20 (2×10), therefore, 95% of the scores in population A will fall between 100 and 60. For population B with scores of 60

± 15, two standard deviations equal 30 (2 × 15), therefore, 95% of the scores in population B will fall between 90 and 30. Values between 60 and 90 could come from either population, reflecting the large overlap that exists between them (Fig. 6-1).

It is important to realize that this discussion of overlap between groups assumes that the populations are distributed in a bell-shaped or normal (Gaussian) distribution. Many measurements on human populations do not follow this distribution. However, regardless of the distribution of the population, statistical theory has shown that at least 75% of all values will be within two standard deviations of the average, and that at least 88% will lie within three standard deviations. Therefore, despite the shape of the distribution, it is possible to get some idea of the overlap of the groups by knowing the averages and the standard deviation. The importance of the degree of overlap between populations is illustrated in the following example.

A study of the white blood cell counts in 10,000 viral infections and 10,000 bacterial infections obtained the following results. Viral infections were associated with white counts of 8,000 ± 500, while bacterial infections were associated with white counts of 9,000 ± 500. Both populations exhibited bell-shaped distributions of values. The results were statistically significant at the .05 level. The authors concluded that a white blood cell count would be an extremely useful means of distinguishing between viral and bacterial infections in the vast majority of cases.

When the reviewer calculates the boundaries of two standard deviations, this conclusion is brought into serious question. If both populations are distributed in a bell-shaped curve, then 95% of the viral infections will have a white count between 7,000 and 9,000, while 95% of the bacterial infections will have a white count between 8,000 and 10,000. Nearly half of the individuals in both groups will have values between 8,000 and 9,000 (Fig. 6-2). In the 8,000 to 9,000 range the values are of little clinical usefulness in distinguishing viral from bacterial infections. Despite the statistical significance of the finding, the large degree of the overlap of values limits its clinical usefulness.

Figure 6-3 demonstrates the thought process that goes into deciding whether one has obtained a clinically important difference and indicates that statistical methods do not always identify true differences. Even when true differences are identified, only a por-

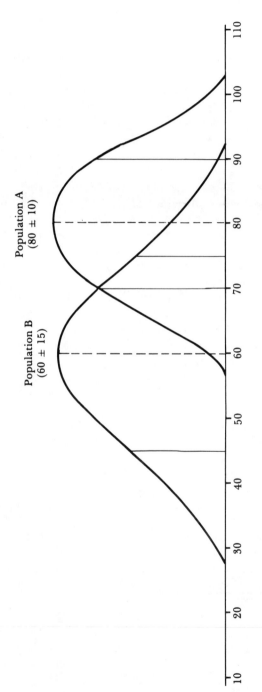

FIGURE 6-1. Overlap that may occur between two groups even in the presence of a statistically significant difference between the mean or the average values. Dotted lines indicate mean values, while the solid, vertical lines indicate one standard deviation from the mean.

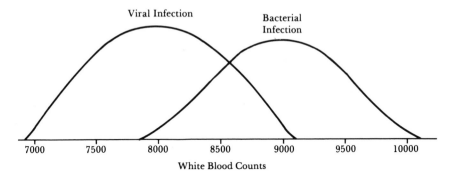

FIGURE 6-2. Degree of overlap between viral and bacterial white blood cell counts even in the presence of a statistically significant difference between the mean or average values.

tion of these will be clinically useful. It even is possible to fail to demonstrate statistical significance when clinically important differences exist in the larger population. The reader must appreciate the limitations and interpretation of statistical significance. Performance of a statistical significance test, even the correct one, is not the be-all and end-all of research. Not all statistically significant differences are important and not all important differences are statistically significant. However, the use of statistical significance testing, tempered with a look at the data, often provides the insights necessary to reach important conclusions.

Contributory Cause

Can cigarettes cause cancer? Can cholesterol cause coronary artery disease? Can chemicals cause congenital defects? The clinician is constantly confronted with controversies over cause and effect. The reader must have an understanding of the concept of causation used by investigators.

The clinical concept of cause, called contributory cause, is an empirical definition that requires the fulfillment of the following criteria: 1) The characteristic referred to as the cause must be shown to precede the effect; 2) altering only the cause must be shown to alter the effect. It may appear simple to establish that a cause precedes an effect, but let us look at two hypothetical studies in which the authors were fooled into believing that they had established that cause precedes effect.

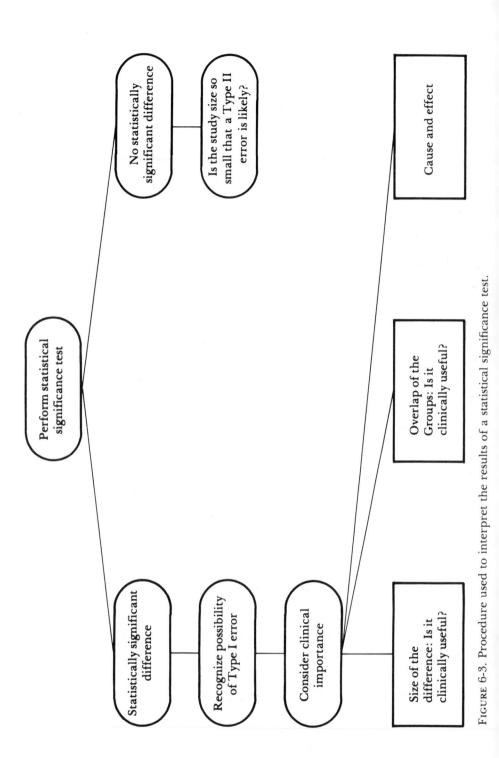

FIGURE 6-3. Procedure used to interpret the results of a statistical significance test.

Two investigators, conducting a retrospective study of drugs taken by patients with myocardial infarction (MI) the week preceding an MI, were looking for the precipitating causes of the condition. Myocardial infarction patients were compared to patients admitted for elective surgery. The authors found that the MI patients were 10 times as likely to have taken aspirin or antacids as the controls during the week preceding admission. The authors concluded that taking aspirin and antacids is associated with subsequent MIs.

The authors believe that they have established the first condition for demonstrating causation, that is, that cause precedes effect. But have they? If individuals have angina prior to MIs, they may misinterpret the pain and try to alleviate it by self-medicating with aspirin or antacids. Therefore, the medication is being taken to treat the disease and does not truly precede the disease. This study failed to establish a prior or antecedent cause because it did not clarify whether the disease led the patients to take the medication or whether the medication precipitated the disease. This example illustrates the frequent difficulty encountered in separating cause and effect in retrospective studies.

Prospective studies have an advantage in establishing that the possible "cause" occurs prior to the "effect." Generally, since the cause (characteristic) is established prior to the occurrence of the effect, the reporting of the cause is not usually affected by knowledge of occurrence of the effect. The following example, however, illustrates that even prospective studies may have difficulty determining whether the cause precedes the effect.

A group of 1,000 patients who had stopped smoking cigarettes within the last year were compared to 1,000 current cigarette smokers matched for total-pack years of smoking. The two groups were followed for 6 months to determine the frequency with which they developed lung cancer. The study showed that 5% of the study group who had stopped smoking cigarettes developed lung cancer as opposed to only 0.1% of the controls. The authors concluded that to stop cigarette smoking was a prior attribute associated with the development of lung cancer. Therefore, they advised current smokers to continue smoking.

The stopping of cigarette smoking appears to occur prior to the development of lung cancer, but what if smokers stop smoking because of symptoms produced by lung cancer? If this were true, then lung cancer stops smoking and not vice versa. Thus, one must be careful in accepting that the hypothesized cause precedes the effect. The ability of prospective studies to establish that cause precedes effect is enhanced when the time lapse between cause and effect is longer than in this example. Short time intervals still leave open the possibility that the cause has been influenced by the effect instead of the reverse.

Even if one has firmly established that the possible cause precedes the effect, it is necessary to establish that altering the cause alters the effect. To understand what is meant and what is not meant by this second requirement, let us look at the following example.

Studies had shown that town X, which took its drinking water from a nearby lake, had five times the subsequent incidence of typhoid fever as that of a similar neighboring town, Y, which used well water. After switching to well water, town X's incidence of typhoid fever fell to the same rate as town Y's. Investigators were disappointed when reviewers of their study concluded that even though the investigation was methodologically proper, the criteria for contributory cause had not been fulfilled. The reviewers argued that there was no explanation of how or why lake water caused typhoid fever so that lake water could not be considered a contributory cause.

If the study was performed properly, these investigators have fulfilled the criteria for contributory cause. Drinking lake water was shown to precede the development of typhoid fever and altering the water supply altered the effect. Remember that contributory cause is an empirical definition. It does not require an intermediate mechanism by which the contributory cause brings about the effect. Historically, there are numerous instances in which actions based on a demonstration of contributory cause reduced disease despite the absence of a scientific understanding of how the result actually occurred. Cholera was controlled through hygiene before its bacterial etiology was understood. Malaria was controlled by swamp clearance before its mosquito transmission was recognized. Scurvy was prevented by citrus fruit before the British ever heard of vitamin C.

Further investigations may be prompted by these studies that may establish the mechanism by which a contributory cause brings about its effect. Prior to understanding the immediate mechanism involved, the adoption of action based on this definition of cause and effect may well be warranted. Investigators, however, must be careful that any change that they observe is not associated with other unobserved changes that are the "real" contributory cause. This pitfall is illustrated by the following example.

In a poor rural community where the diet was very low in protein, diarrhea was widespread. The effect of increased protein was studied in randomly selected areas through the introduction of high protein crops, using modern agricultural methods. Subsequent follow-up revealed a 70% reduction in the incidence of diarrhea in the affected areas with little change in the other areas. The authors concluded that a high protein diet prevents diarrheal disease.

It is likely that the introduction of modern agriculture was associated with numerous other changes in water supply and sanitation that may have contributed as well to the reduced incidences of diarrhea. Thus, even in an experimental study, caution must be observed to be sure that the characteristic selected as the cause is truly the factor that brought about the effect. In other words, the investigator and the reader must be careful that the cause has truly preceded the effect and that the presumed alteration in the effect has not been produced by other changes that are actually causal.

It is important to realize that the contributory cause may be many steps removed from the immediate cause of the disease. This definition, called contributory cause, would have established bad water as the cause of cholera, swamps as the etiology of malaria, and the absence of citrus fruit as the cause of scurvy. Altering these factors may reduce disease even though they have their effect through other more immediate causes. The identification of a contributory cause may be very important to the control of the disease even though much remains to be learned about the immediate biological mechanism for disease production. It may be helpful to review a sequence of studies frequently conducted to establish the existence of a contributory cause.

Researchers often begin with a retrospective study when exploring or "fishing" for possible causes. Retrospective studies have the advantage of speed, low cost, and the ability to study numerous possible causes all at once. The retrospective method aims to establish the existence of associations or relationships between factors, but there is more difficulty in establishing that the cause precedes the effect.

Once an association is established in one or more retrospective studies, investigators then frequently proceed to prospective studies. Despite the need for careful interpretation as illustrated in the smoking cessation example, the prospective method is better able to establish that the cause precedes the effect.

Having established that a possible cause precedes the effect, investigators usually turn to the experimental method to establish that altering the cause alters the effect. The true experimental method, in which individuals are randomly and blindly assigned and only the study group is exposed to the possible cause or proposed treatment, is a powerful tool for demonstrating contributory cause. However, because of ethical or logistical considerations, investigators frequently need to rely on "natural experiments" to determine whether altering the cause alters the effect. This sequence of studies might proceed as follows in establishing that estrogen causes uterine cancer.

Not knowing the causes of uterine cancer, investigators might conduct a retrospective study exploring numerous hypotheses, including an association between estrogens and uterine cancer. If an association is found, the investigators then would conduct a prospective study to more firmly establish that taking estrogens precedes uterine cancer. They would want to be sure that estrogens are not given to treat any bleeding that could be a symptom of cancer. The prospective study would establish similar groups of patients who can be observed while taking or not taking estrogens over a period of time. The investigators would determine whether the estrogen-taking group develops more uterine cancer than the group not taking estrogen. The prospective study may more firmly establish that taking estrogens precedes the subsequent development of uterine cancer.

Often, however, a prospective study is considered too expensive or too time-consuming and the evidence that cause precedes effect must come entirely from retrospective studies. When one is restricted to retrospective studies, it is often helpful to determine whether the association is consistent and dose-related. That is, does the risk of disease increase with increased duration of dosage exposure and does it hold up in other studies conducted on different populations?

Having provided suggestive evidence that estrogens are dangerous, however, it might be unethical to conduct a controlled clinical trial of the relationship between estrogens and uterine cancer. Investigators may be forced to look for natural experiments to confirm that estrogens are a contributory cause of uterine cancer. Such a natural experiment may occur, for instance, if one population discontinues estrogen use as a result of the publicity generated by the studies. If the population that discontinued estrogen use experiences a declining uterine cancer rate not found in a group that continues estrogen use, this natural experiment may provide evidence that altering the cause alters the effect. Thus retrospective, prospective, and experimental studies all may play a role in establishing the criteria for contributory cause.

Other Concepts of Causation

The concept of contributory cause has been a very useful concept in studying disease. Contributory cause, however, is not the only concept of causation that has been used in clinical medicine. In the 19th century, Robert Koch developed a series of conditions that needed to be fulfilled before a microorganism could be considered the cause of a disease. The conditions known as *Koch's postulate* included requirements that the organism is always found with the disease, and that the organism is not found with any other disease.

These conditions represent additional requirements beyond those necessary for establishing contributory cause. Historically, these were very useful in the study of infectious disease in circumstances where a single agent is responsible for a single disease. However, if Koch's postulate is applied to the study of chronic diseases, it is nearly impossible to prove a causal relationship. For instance, even though cigarettes have been carefully established as a contributory cause of lung cancer, cigarettes are not always found in association with lung cancer. In addition, cigarettes may contribute to coronary artery disease and laryngeal cancer and thus may well be found with other diseases. Even with infectious disease, Koch's postulate may be too strict to be clinically useful. For instance, mononucleosis is a well-established clinical illness that has been shown to have the Barr-Epstein virus as a contributory cause. However, other viruses such as cytomegalovirus also have been shown to bring about the mononucleosis syndrome. In addition, the Barr-Epstein virus, under the right circumstances, has been shown to be a contributory cause of a cancer known as Birkett's lymphoma. Thus, despite the fact that the Barr-Epstein virus has been established as a contributory cause of the mononucleosis syndrome, neither of Koch's fundamental postulates have been fulfilled.

In formal logic, Koch's postulate that the organism is always found with the disease is known as *necessary cause*. This rule implies that if the cause is absent so is the disease (for instance: no cigarettes, no lung cancer). Under the rules of strict logic, causation requires a second condition known as *sufficient cause*. This condition says that if the cause is present so is the disease. For instance, if cigarette smoking occurs, so will lung cancer. The next example illustrates the consequences of applying the necessary cause of formal logic to medical studies.

In a study of the risk factors for coronary artery disease, investigators identified 100 individuals from a population of 10,000 MI patients who have experienced MIs despite normal blood pressure, normal cholesterol, regular exercise, no smoking, Type B personality, and no family history of coronary artery disease. The authors concluded that they had demonstrated that hypertension, high cholesterol, lack of exercise, smoking, Type A personality, and family history were not the causes of coronary artery disease since not every MI patient possessed a risk factor.

The authors of this study were using the necessary cause of formal logic as a concept of cause. Instead of necessary cause, however, let us assume that all these factors had been shown to fulfill the criteria for contributory cause of coronary artery disease. Contributory cause, unlike necessary cause, does not require that all those who are free of the cause will be free of the effect. The failure of known contributory cause to predict all the cases of disease emphasizes the limitations of our current knowledge about all the contributory causes of coronary artery disease. It illustrates our current state of ignorance, for if all the contributory causes were known, then all those with disease would possess at least one such factor. Thus even when a contributory cause has been established, it does not imply that it will necessarily be present in each and every case. The following example illustrates the consequences of applying formal logic's criteria of sufficient cause.

In a study of a new strain of meningococcal virus in the military, 10,000 healthy men were identified as being infected with the new organism. Using random assignment, half the men were assigned to a treatment group and half were assigned to a placebo group. Among the treated patients, none developed meningitis during the next 12 months, while 5% of the placebo group developed meningitis infection from the new organism. The authors concluded that a cause and effect relationship had not been established since most of the untreated patients did not develop meningitis.

These authors adopted the criteria of sufficient cause from formal logic, that is, the mere presence of the cause must always be associated with the effect. Even in infectious disease situations, a contributory cause may not always lead to the effect. The authors of the study did establish that the new organism is a prior attribute and that eliminating the cause eliminates the effect. They therefore have provided adequate proof to establish the new organism as a contributory cause even if the criteria of sufficient cause is not fulfilled.

In summary, the clinically useful definition of causation is known as contributory cause. It requires a demonstration that the presumed cause precedes the effect, and that altering the cause alters the effect. It does not require that all those who possess the contributory cause necessarily will develop the effect. It does not require that all those who are free of the contributory cause will be free of the effect. In other words, a clinical cause may be neither necessary nor sufficient, but it must be contributory.

Previous chapters have illustrated the errors that can be made in assigning patients to study and control groups, assessing a study outcome, and analyzing and interpreting the results of a study. Having completed this process, the investigator now asks what meaning all this has for individuals not included in the study. To obtain the meaning of the study for the larger, outside population, the investigator must extrapolate the results of the study to new and potentially different situations.

It is no easier to escape the errors of extrapolation than to avoid the errors of assignment, assessment, analysis, or interpretation. There are four types of errors in extrapolating the study results to the larger population:

1. Errors in extrapolating beyond the range of the data
2. Errors in extrapolating from population data to conclusions about individuals
3. Errors resulting from unappreciated factors in a new population
4. Errors in extrapolating from the study population to the general population

Beyond the Range of the Data

In clinical studies, individuals are exposed to the factors thought to be associated with the outcome for only a limited amount of time at a limited range of exposure. The investigators may be studying a factor such as hypertension that results in a stroke or a therapeutic agent such as cimetadine that is associated with the healing of an ulcer. In either case, the interpretation must be limited to the range and duration of hypertension experienced by the subjects or the dosage and duration of cimetadine employed in the study. When the investigators draw conclusions that go beyond the duration and range experienced by the study subjects, they frequently are making unwarranted assumptions. They may assume that longer exposure will continue to produce the same effect experienced by the study subjects. The following example illustrates a potential error resulting from extrapolating beyond the range of the data.

A new antihypertensive agent was tested on 100 resistant hypertensives. It was found to lower diastolic blood pressure in all 100 resistant hypertensives from 120 to 110 at doses of 1 mg per kilogram and from 110 to 100 at doses of 2 mg per kilogram. The authors concluded that this agent would be able to lower diastolic blood pressure from 100 to 90 at doses of 3 mg per kilogram.

It is possible that clinical evidence would document the new agent's efficacy at 3 mg per kg. Such documentation, however, awaits empirical proof. Many antihypertensive agents have been shown to reach maximum effectiveness at a certain dose and not to increase their effectiveness at higher doses. To conclude that higher doses produce greater effects without experimental evidence is to extrapolate beyond the range of the data.

Another type of error associated with extrapolation beyond the range of the data concerns potential side effects experienced at increased exposure, as can be seen in the following hypothetical example.

A one-year study of the effects of administering daily estrogen to 100 menopausal women found that the drug relieved hot flashes and reduced the rate of osteoporosis as opposed to the lack of relief of symptoms in age-matched women given placebos. The authors found no adverse effects from the estrogens and concluded that estrogens are safe and effective. Therefore they recommended that estrogens be administered long-term to women, beginning at the onset of menopause.

The authors have extrapolated from a one-year period of follow-up to long-term administration of estrogens. There is no evidence presented that women either need or would benefit from long-term administration. In addition, there is no evidence to show that if one year of administration is safe, so is long-term, continuous administration of estrogen. It is not likely that any long-term adverse effects would show up in a one-year study. Thus, the authors have made potentially dangerous extrapolations by going beyond the range of their data.

From Populations to Individuals

The second type of extrapolation error involves extrapolating from population data to conclusions about individuals. Medical studies may be conducted using data from separate individuals or by using population data. Studies done by investigators using population data are known as ecological studies. When using group or population data, the investigators frequently have little information about the individuals who make up the population. This lack of individual data may lead investigators to commit the extrapolation error known as ecological fallacy, as illustrated in the following example.

A population study demonstrated that the rate of stomach cancer in Iceland is four times that in the United States. The study data also demonstrated that in Iceland, fish are eaten at a rate four times that of the United States. The authors concluded that eating fish is associated with stomach cancer.

In order to establish an association, the authors must show that those who eat more fish are more likely to develop stomach cancer. Relying on population figures alone does not provide any information about the cause and effect relationship experienced by individuals. It is possible that among the Icelandic population it is the nonfish eaters who get stomach cancer. If this were true, the authors would have committed an ecological fallacy. The establishment of an association between eating fish and developing stomach cancer requires a demonstration that the relationship holds on an individual level.

Another type of error committed in extrapolating from population to individual causation is illustrated in the following hypothetical study.

In a population study of both Japanese society and American society, the Japanese were found to have a 20% prevalence of hypertension and an 80% prevalence of cigarette smoking. Americans were found to have a 10% prevalence of hypertension and a 40% prevalence of cigarette smoking. Despite having twice the prevalence of hypertension and cigarette smoking, the Japanese were found to have only one-tenth the rate of myocardial infarctions. The authors concluded that hypertension and cigarette smoking must protect the Japanese from myocardial infarctions.

The authors have extrapolated from data based on populations to conclusions about individual causation. Other explanations for the observed data are possible. If Americans frequently possess another risk factor, such as a high cholesterol count, which is rare in Japan, this factor may override cigarette smoking and hypertension and help to produce the high rate of myocardial infarctions in the American population.

Unappreciated Factors in a New Population

A third type of extrapolation error occurs when valid data from one study are extrapolated to a population in which unappreciated factors are at work. Without realizing it, the authors may assume that the new population is identical to their study groups. An example of this danger of extrapolating to a new population is illustrated in the following hypothetical study.

A study of the preventive effect of treating borderline tuberculosis (TB) skin tests (6-10 mm) with a year of isoniazid was conducted among Alaskan Eskimos. The population had a prevalence of borderline skin tests of 2 per 1,000. The study was conducted by giving isoniazid to 200 Eskimos with borderline skin tests and placebos to 200 other Eskimos with the same borderline condition. There were 20 cases of active TB among the placebo patients and only one among the patients given isoniazid. The results were statistically significant at the .05 level. A health official from Georgia where borderline skin tests occur in 300 per 1,000 skin tests was very impressed with these results. He advocated treating all Georgian patients who had borderline skin tests with isoniazid for one year.

In extrapolating to the Georgian population, the health official has assumed that borderline skin tests meant the same among Alaskan Eskimos as among the Georgia population. Other data suggest, however, that many borderline skin tests in Georgia are not due to TB exposure. Instead of indicating TB, they are frequently caused by an atypical mycobacteria that carries a much more benign prognosis and does not reliably respond to isoniazid. The health official has ignored the fact that borderline skin tests have a very different meaning among Eskimos compared to residents of Georgia. By not appreciating this new factor in the residents of Georgia, the health official may be submitting large numbers of individuals to useless and potentially dangerous therapy.

From Study Population to General Population

The fourth type of extrapolation error occurs when valid results from a study population are applied directly to the general population without taking into account the frequency of the condition in the general population. It is important to distinguish the degree of risk observed in a study from the degree of risk in the general population. The risk among the study population is known as the *relative* risk. It measures the risk in the study group versus the risk in the control group. When applying this risk to the general population, one asks what proportion of the disease in the general population is attributable to the factor under study. This proportion is known as the *attributable* risk.

A large relative risk for a rare characteristic may account for only a small attributable risk in the general population. Conversely, if a study factor is very common in the general population, a small or moderate-sized relative risk in the study may result in a quite large attributable risk in the general population. The need to distinguish relative risk and attributable risk is emphasized in the following examples.

Investigators report that the hereditary form of high cholesterol, known as Type 2 hyperlipidemia, occurs in 1 per 100,000 Americans. They also report that these individuals have 20 times the risk of developing coronary artery disease, versus age- and sex-matched individuals with normal cholesterol. In a well performed, controlled clinical trial, the authors found that a new treatment completely eliminated the risk of coronary artery disease in those with Type 2 hyperlipidemia. They concluded that a widespread application of the treatment to those with Type 2 hyperlipidemia would have a major impact on the national rate of coronary artery disease.

In this instance, investigators assembled a study group made up entirely of Type 2 hyperlipidemia patients. However, they extrapolated their conclusion to the general population in which Type 2 hyperlipidemia is rare. Therefore, even if the risk of the disease were eliminated by the new treatment, it would have little effect on the overall rate of coronary artery disease since Type 2 hyperlipidemia is such a rare condition. This study illustrates the occurrence of a large relative risk that results only in a small attributable risk when applied to the general population.

While the previous example illustrated how a successful treatment can appear less important when extrapolated to the general population, the following example illustrates that the reverse can also be true.

A long-term experimental study randomly assigned age-matched, middle-aged men to both an exercise group and a nonexercise group. It was found that men in the exercise group performed three times the amount of exercise as the nonexercise group. In this well-controlled study, those in the exercise group had 10% fewer MIs as compared to the nonexercise group. The authors concluded that the very small reduction in the risk of MIs in the study meant that exercise could have little overall effect on MIs in the general population.

In this case, the relative reduction in risk is much smaller than in the previous example. However, exercise is a characteristic potentially applicable to nearly the entire population that risks having MIs. A 10% reduction in risk, when applied to a large population, would result in a large number of prevented MIs. Thus, in extrapolating the results of a study to the general population, the authors must consider not only the relative reduction in risk in their study population, but also the extent to which their results can be applied to the general population.

This example illustrates how a small to moderate decrease in relative risk can result in a quite large reduction in the occurrence of the disease in the general population.

Having completed our discussion of the requirements for proper implementation of the components of the uniform framework, let us go back to the beginning and ask some basic questions.

1. Were the aims of the study adequately defined?
2. Were the study hypotheses clearly delineated?
3. What is the study type? Is it appropriate to the questions being asked?
4. What is the study population? Is it adequate to answer the study questions?

The answers to these questions will tell the reader whether the investigators have chosen an appropriate study design, that is, one that defines and addresses the intended study questions.

Aim of the Study

Investigators may desire to study the end-organ effects of hypertension but the inability to perform renal biopsies and cerebral angiograms may force them to carefully study retinal changes. Researchers may wish to investigate the long-term effects of a new drug to prevent osteoporosis, but time, money, and the desire to publish may limit their investigation to its short-term effects on bone metabolism and bone density. It is essential that the investigators and the reader distinguish between what the investigators ideally would like to study and what they are in fact studying.

Clarifying the Hypothesis

When studying end-organ damage due to hypertension, the investigators' hypothesis should not be that the degree of end-organ damage will correlate with the degree of hypertension, but rather that the degree of narrowing of the retinal arteries will correlate with the degree of hypertension. The latter formulation provides a specific study question that can be addressed by an investigation.

Failure to clarify the hypotheses being tested makes it difficult for the researcher and for the reader to choose and assess the study design. It also makes it more difficult in the end to determine whether the aims of the study have been achieved. Finally, as was pointed out in our discussion of statistical significance testing, without prior formulation of specific hypotheses the usual tests of statistical significance are not applicable.

Identifying the Study Type

Having defined the specific study hypotheses, the reader is ready to identify the type of study that was performed and to evaluate the appropriateness of the type chosen. There is rarely only one type of study design that is appropriate to a study question. At times, however, the disadvantages of one type of study design may make it very difficult to accomplish the study aims. In order to help the reader judge the appropriateness of a chosen study design, let us outline the advantages and disadvantages of our basic types of studies.

RETROSPECTIVE STUDIES

Retrospective or case-control studies have the distinct advantage of being able to study rare conditions or diseases. If the condition is rare, retrospective studies are able to detect differences between groups using far fewer individuals. The time required to perform a retrospective study is often much less than for a prospective study, since the disease has already developed. The retrospective method allows investigators to explore simultaneously the possible multiple associations with a disease. One could explore, for instance, the many variables that possibly are associated with colon cancer. Prior diet, surgery, ulcerative colitis, polyps, alcohol, cigarettes, family history, and many other variables all might be investigated in the same study.

The major objection to retrospective studies is that they are prone to the variety of methodological errors that were illustrated in the hypothetical studies. Many of the errors involve the accuracy of the data about the prior characteristics. The retrospective method is often an excellent method for establishing a prior association especially when there is no reason to believe that the researcher's or the study subject's knowledge of the presence of a disease affects the assessment of past data.

PROSPECTIVE STUDIES

Prospective studies have the major advantage of greater assurance that the characteristic under study preceded the outcome under study. This is a critical distinction when assessing a cause and effect relationship. Concurrent prospective studies, which follow patients forward over long periods of time, are expensive and time-consuming. It is possible, however, to perform a prospective study without such lengthy periods of time. If reliable data on the presence or absence of the study characteristic are available from an earlier time, this data can be used to perform a non-concurrent prospective study. In a non-concurrent prospective study, the assignment of individuals to groups is made on the basis of this past data. The individuals then can be followed forward in time and their subsequent development of disease can be assessed.

For instance, if cholesterol readings were available on a group of young adults from 15 years before the current study began, the patients could be followed forward in time to assess the subsequent development of coronary artery disease, strokes or other consequences of high cholesterol that could occur soon after the time the study begins. The critical element, which characterizes a prospective study, is the assignment of individuals to study and control groups before the disease or condition under study has developed.

Since prospective studies are able to delineate the various types of effects caused by an agent already expected to cause at least one condition, the researcher can study simultaneously the relationship between hypertension and stroke, myocardial infarction, heart failure, and renal disease. Prospective studies can produce more in-depth understanding of the effect of an etiological factor but they are less likely than retrospective studies to uncover new etiological factors.

EXPERIMENTAL STUDIES

Both retrospective and prospective studies are observational, that is, they observe the characteristics and outcomes of individuals rather than impose the characteristics. Experimental studies are distinguished from observational studies by the intervention that occurs when an investigator randomly and blindly assigns individuals to groups. The ability to assign individuals helps to assure that it is the study characteristic and not some underlying predisposition that links the study characteristic with the outcome. The ability to impose intervention on one group also helps to establish cause and effect relationships by determining that altering the cause alters the effect.

Intervention can be accomplished in a clinical trial in which a randomly and blindly assigned study group receives a treatment while a comparable control group is given a placebo. The investigator then is able to determine whether the treatment that alters the cause results in an altered effect.

CROSS-SECTIONAL STUDIES
The three basic types of studies discussed here are not the only types of studies one will encounter in the medical literature. Cross-sectional studies also are frequently performed. In these investigations the study characteristic and the outcome are measured at the same point in time, in other words, the assignment and assessment are measured simultaneously. Cross-sectional studies are useful when one expects that continued exposure is required right up to the time that the disease develops. When studying thrombophlebitis and its relationship to birth control pills, one might use a cross-sectional study. One would study whether women with thrombophlebitis are more likely to be on birth control pills at the time they develop thrombophlebitis than a comparable group of women without thrombophlebitis. Except for the assessment of outcome concurrently with the assignment, cross-sectional studies are identical to retrospective studies.

Composition of the Study Sample
Having defined the study aims, the study hypothesis and the study type, the reader should then concentrate on the sample of individuals selected for study. The reader should ask the following questions:

1. Do the individuals selected come from a population capable of addressing the study hypothesis?
2. Are there an adequate number of patients to allow reasonable chance of demonstrating a difference between the groups?

In examining the population from which the study sample was selected, the reader needs to keep the hypothesis carefully in mind. Failure to relate the study population to the hypothesis can lead to the following type of error.

Investigators wish to test a new therapy designed to prevent chronic smokers from developing lung cancer by strengthening their immune system. They select 1,000 heavy smokers with lung cancer and randomly and blindly assign 500 to the new treatment and 500 to a placebo group. They find that there is no difference in the survival of the two groups. They conclude that their study refutes the value of the new therapy for preventing lung cancer.

The researchers have chosen a group of patients who already have developed the disease, which they desire to prevent. They have apparently forgotten that they sought to study the new treatment's potential for preventing the disease; therefore, their study sample is not properly chosen to test their hypothesis. Even if the study implementation is perfect, the inherent design of the study is incapable of answering the proposed study question. Failure to demonstrate a difference between groups does not add evidence for or against the researcher's hypothesis. Generally the errors that can occur in actual studies are more subtle, but the principle of relating the study hypothesis to the study design is important for assessing the adequacy of the study.

Size of the Study Sample

Having addressed the study aims, the study hypothesis, the study types, and the composition of the study sample, it is helpful to have a means of judging the adequacy of the sample size. The reader should be aware of the size of the true difference between the outcome both in the study and the control groups, which is likely to produce statistically significant results in an investigation.

In addressing the question of adequacy of sample size, we need to distinguish between cross-sectional and retrospective studies on the one hand and prospective and experimental studies on the other hand. Remember that in cross-sectional and retrospective studies the outcome is a characteristic of the patient, while in prospective and experimental studies the outcome is the disease. Thus in retrospective and cross-sectional studies, one is interested in how small a difference in a patient characteristic (such as use of birth control pills) is likely to be shown to be statistically significant, given the sample size used in the study. In prospective or experimental studies, one is interested in how small a difference in the probability of developing a disease (such as a stroke) is likely to be shown to be statistically significant, given the sample size used in the study.

Answers to these questions depend on the size of the Type I and Type II errors that the reader and investigator are willing to tolerate. Remember that a Type I error is the probability of demonstrating a statistically significant difference when no true difference exists in the larger populations from which the study and control groups are sampled. A Type II error is the probability of failing to demonstrate a statistically significant difference when a true difference actually does exist in the larger populations from which the study and control groups are sampled.

The Type I error that will be tolerated is usually set at 5%. This is traditional and arbitrary, but it is consistent with the 5% level of uncertainty widely used in statistics. The Type II error that will be tolerated is open for discussion. Most investigators would like the probability of failing to demonstrate the statistical significance of a true difference to be 10% or less. The sizes of the true differences in outcome for which one can expect to demonstrate a statistically significant difference are as follows. We will assume a 5% Type I error and a 10% Type II error and apply standard statistical tables.*

1. If 100 individuals are included in the study group and 100 in the control group, a difference in outcome of 25% or more is likely to be demonstrated as statistically significant.
2. If the study group and the control group each contain 250 individuals, than a 15% or greater difference in outcome can be expected to produce results that are statistically significant.
3. In order to expect to show statistical significance for true differences of only 10% or more, over 550 individuals should be included in both the study and control groups.
4. The ability to demonstrate statistical significance for differences of 5% or more between the study group and the control group requires over 2,000 individuals in each group.

If the investigators can make separate estimates of the outcome both in the study and control groups, they can be more accurate in estimating how small a true difference they are likely to detect.

*Fleiss, J. L. *Statistical Methods for Rates and Proportions.* New York: Wiley, 1973, p. 190.

At times they may be able to detect differences smaller than indicated here.

Let us now apply these principles of sample size to demonstrate why retrospective studies or cross-sectional studies are useful for studying rare diseases that affect relatively small numbers of individuals. Remember that the term *outcome* refers to a characteristic of the patient in cross-sectional and retrospective studies, and to the disease itself in prospective and experimental studies. The following hypothetical study shows the difficulty in demonstrating statistical significance when a prospective study is used to investigate a rare disease.

Investigators wished to study whether birth control pills are associated with the rare occurrence of strokes in young women. The researchers followed 20,000 women on birth control pills and 20,000 women on other forms of birth control for 10 years. After spending millions of dollars in follow-up, they found two cases of stroke among the pill users and one case among the nonpill users. The differences were not statistically significant. Despite the small number of stroke patients that they found, the investigators concluded that at least they had used an infallible prospective study rather than a worthless retrospective study.

When a disease is very rare, such as strokes in young women, it often requires enormous numbers of individuals to demonstrate a statistically significant difference if a prospective study is used. Assume, for instance, that the rate of strokes among young women not on the pill is 1 per 100,000 or .001%. Let us further assume that birth control pills increase this risk ten fold to 1 per 10,000 or .01%. The difference in outcome is thus .01% − .001% or .009%. The use of a prospective study to demonstrate a statistically significant difference for a true difference this small may require well over 100,000 women in each group.

On the other hand, if a retrospective study is performed using young women with strokes as the study group and young women without strokes as the control group, the outcome being measured is now the use of birth control pills rather than strokes. Groups of 250 each will then be adequate for detecting a statistically significant difference if there actually is a 15% difference in the use of birth control pills between women with strokes and women without strokes. In this instance, it is feasible to perform a retrospective study of the relationship between birth control pills and strokes, using only a small fraction of the individuals required to study the same question with a prospective study. Therefore this prospective study was doomed to failure from the beginning; a retrospective study would have been far more appropriate.

Whenever an investigation fails to demonstrate a statistically significant difference, the reader must appreciate the size of the true difference between groups that one would expect to detect given the number of individuals both in the study and control groups. An understanding of study design also requires the reader to appreciate the aims of the study, the specific study hypothesis being tested, the study type being employed, and the study population chosen. Equipped with an understanding of these basic issues, the reader can evaluate the results of the study more intelligently.

Studying a Study

Study Design

In determining whether the study was properly designed to answer the study questions, the reviewer must initially determine whether the study aims were sufficiently defined. Then the reader should ask whether an appropriate study population was chosen to answer the study questions. Finally, the critical reader must take into account the advantages and disadvantages of each type of study to determine whether the study type chosen was appropriate to the questions being asked.

Assignment

Investigators attempt to assemble study and control groups that are identical in all respects except for the characteristic(s) under study. Retrospective and prospective studies are susceptible to the assignment error of selection bias that occurs whenever study or control groups are not representative of all individuals who could have been included and this uniqueness affects the outcome of the study. All the four types of study design may result in noncomparability whenever there are chance differences between the study and control groups that are related to the study outcome. When noncomparable groups occur it is important that the reader recognize this fact so that adjustment for these differences can be made in the analysis.

Assessment

In assessing the outcome of a study, the reviewer must consider whether the requirements for a valid assessment have been fulfilled. The investigators must show that they have chosen an appropriate measure of outcome, one that measures what they intended to measure. They must have performed an accurate assessment, that is, a precise and complete evaluation. Finally, they must have considered whether the process of observation affected the outcome of the study.

Analysis

Before comparing the study and control groups, investigators must show they have taken into account the differences between the study and control groups. In comparing the outcomes for the study and control groups, investigators also must show they have calculated the size of the difference and applied a test of statistical significance. These tests determine the probability that the results could have occurred by chance. Study data are often presented showing the averages of the groups plus standard deviations. These measures of variability within the study and control groups help to determine the degree of overlap between them.

Interpretation

The authors of a study must demonstrate that they have asked what the results mean for those included in the study. They ask whether the probability of the results occurring by chance is small enough for the null hypothesis to be rejected and, by elimination, the study hypothesis accepted. They then ask whether the size of the differences and the degree of overlap is such that the results are clinically useful or important. Finally, they ask whether the criteria for a cause and effect relationship have been established. They apply the clinical concept of contributory cause.

Contributory cause requires that the presumed cause precedes the effect and that altering the cause alters the effect. It does not require that the cause is necessary or sufficient to produce the effect.

Extrapolation

Finally the investigators must ask what the study results mean for those not included in the study. In extrapolating to new populations or new situations they must avoid going beyond the data. They must beware of the ecological fallacies which may occur when extrapolating from population data to individuals. They must also consider altered underlying assumptions and differences in prevalence between the study population and the general population.

Few investigations are free of all these errors; however, their presence does not automatically invalidate an investigation. It is the responsibility of the critical reader to recognize the errors and take them into account when applying the results of the study.

Questions to Ask in Studying a Study

Let us now put the foregoing material together and see if you can apply what you have learned to simulated research articles. The critical method for evaluating a research study is outlined in the following checklist of questions to ask when you are studying a study.

1. Study Design: Was the study properly designed?
   a. Were the aims of the study sufficiently defined?
   b. Were the study hypotheses clearly delineated?
   c. What was the study type? Was it appropriate to the questions being asked?
   d. What was the study population? Was it of adequate composition and size to answer the study questions?
2. Assignment: Was the assignment of patients to study and control groups proper?
   a. If the study was retrospective or prospective, could selection bias have occurred?
   b. If the study was experimental, was random and blind assignment maintained?
   c. Regardless of the study type, were the study and control groups comparable with respect to characteristics other than the study factor(s)?
3. Assessment: Was the assessment of outcome properly performed in the study and the control groups?
   a. Was the measure of outcome appropriate to the study aims?
   b. Was the measure of outcome precise?
   c. Was the measure of outcome complete?
   d. Did the process of observation affect the outcome?
4. Analysis: Did the analysis properly compare the outcomes in the study and the control groups?
   a. Were the results adjusted to take into account the effect of possible confounding variables?
   b. Was a significance test properly performed to assess the probability that the difference was due to chance?

    c. Was a proper measure of the size of the difference presented?

    d. Was a proper measure of the degree of overlap of the differences presented?

5. Interpretation: Was a valid interpretation drawn from the comparisons made between the study and control groups during analysis?

    a. Did the investigators properly reject or fail to reject the null hypothesis?

    b. Did the investigators consider the possibility of Type I and Type II errors in interpreting the meaning of the significance test?

    c. Were the size of the differences and the degree of overlap taken into consideration in the conclusions reached about the meaning of observed differences?

    d. In interpreting the meaning of any relationship, was the clinical concept of cause and effect (contributory cause) properly applied?

6. Extrapolation: Were the extrapolations to individuals not included in the study properly performed?

    a. Did the investigators stay within the limits of the data when extrapolating the results?

    b. If the investigators extrapolated from population data to individual data, did they commit an ecological fallacy?

    c. Did the researchers take into consideration differences between the study population and the population to which they extrapolated their data?

The following hypothetical studies include errors of the type illustrated in each of the components of the basic framework. These flaw-catching exercises are designed to test your ability to apply the basic framework in order to critically study a study. Examples of retrospective, prospective, and experimental studies are presented. Please read the exercises and, using the outline, write a critique of each study. A sample critique that points out important errors follows each exercise.

Note that the final flaw-catching exercise is the same one you read at the beginning of the book. Compare your current critique of this review exercise to the one you wrote previously to see how much progress you have made.

Exercise No. 1: Retrospective Study

A retrospective investigation was undertaken in order to study the factors associated with the development of congenital heart disease (CHD) in fetuses. Two hundred women with first-trimester, spontaneous abortions in which congenital heart abnormalities were found in the fetus upon pathological examination were used as the study group. The control group was composed of 200 women with consecutive, first-trimester, induced abortions in which no congenital heart defects were found.

An attempt was made to interview each one of the 400 women within one month after her abortion to determine which factors in the pregnancy may have led to CHD. One hundred different variables were studied. The interviewers gained the participation of 120 of the 200 study group women who experienced spontaneous abortions and 80 of the 200 control group women who underwent induced abortions. The other women refused to participate in the study.

The investigators found the following differences between women whose fetuses had CHD and those whose fetuses were not affected:

1. Women with CHD fetuses were three times as likely to use antinausea medications during pregnancy as women whose fetuses did not have CHD. The difference was statistically significant at the .05 level.

2. There was no difference in the use of tranquilizers between the study group and the control group.
3. Women with CHD fetuses had an average age of 23 years versus 18 years for women whose fetuses did not have CHD. The results were statistically significant.
4. The women with CHD fetuses drank an average of 3.7 cups of coffee per day, while women whose fetuses did not have CHD drank an average of 3.5 cups of coffee per day. The differences were statistically significant.
5. Among the other 96 variables studied, the authors found that women with CHD fetuses were twice as likely to have blond hair and to be over 5 ft. 6 in. tall. Both differences were statistically significant using the usual statistical methods.

The authors drew the following conclusions:

1. Antinausea medications cause CHD since they are more often used by women whose fetuses have CHD.
2. Tranquilizers are safe for use in pregnancy since they were not associated with an increased risk of CHD.
3. Since women in their twenties are more likely to have fetuses with CHD, women should be encouraged to have their children before age 20.
4. Since coffee drinking increases the risk of CHD, coffee drinking should be eliminated completely during pregnancy, which would largely eliminate the risk of CHD.
5. Despite the fact that no one had hypothesized height and hair color as risk factors for CHD, these were proven to be important predictors of CHD.

Critique: Exercise No. 1
STUDY DESIGN
The investigators have not clarified the aims of their study. Are they interested in specific types of CHD? Congential heart disease consists of a variety of conditions involving valves, septum, and blood vessels. In lumping all conditions under the heading CHD, the investigators are assuming that there is a common etiology for all these conditions. In addition, the specific hypotheses being tested are not clarified in this study. The populations chosen consist

of a study group who underwent spontaneous abortion and a control group who underwent voluntary induced abortions. These groups can be expected to be different in a variety of ways. It would have been preferable to choose more comparable groups of women, for instance, those who had induced abortions with and without CHD or who had spontaneous abortions with and without CHD.

With this study design it must be remembered that only CHD that was severe enough to cause early spontaneous abortion is being studied. While this may provide important information, the factors causing CHD severe enough to abort fetuses may be different from the factors causing CHD in full term babies.

ASSIGNMENT
To determine whether a selection bias exists, we ask, first, if the study group and the control group differ in some respect. Secondly, we ask if these differences have affected the results. The experiences of women having induced abortions versus women having spontaneous abortions are likely to be different in many ways. It is probable that the women also have different attitudes about their pregnancies, which may affect their use of drugs during pregnancy. Such differences between the study group and the control group could affect the results so that selection bias may well be present.

ASSESSMENT
The high rate of loss of participants to follow-up suggests the possibility that those who did participate in the study had different attributes from those who did not. A high rate of loss to follow-up weakens the conclusions that can be drawn from any observed differences. Biased recall on the part of the participants is a possibility, particularly when the subject matter has a high emotional content. The retrospective reporting of drug use may be especially influenced by the emotions surrounding the loss of the fetus among those experiencing an unwanted, spontaneous abortion. The result may be a closer scrutiny of the memory, leading to a more thorough recall of drug use.

ANALYSIS, INTERPRETATION, AND EXTRAPOLATION
1. Even if one assumes that the relationship between antinausea medications and CHD was properly derived, it has not been shown

that a cause and effect relationship exists. Retrospective studies cannot definitively settle the question of which factor is the "cause" and which is the "effect." It is possible that women with CHD fetuses have more nausea and therefore take more antinausea medications. Before a causal relationship is established in the clinical sense of causation (contributory cause), investigators must show that the postulated cause precedes the effect and that altering the cause alters the effect. The authors of this study have drawn an interpretation that is not necessarily warranted by the data. Adjusting the analysis for prevalence of nausea during pregnancy would be one method to further evaluate the possible relationship between antinausea medications and CHD while still using a retrospective study.

2. The absence of a difference between groups in terms of use of tranquilizers does not necessarily assure the safety of these drugs. The samples may be too small to fully test the risk of tranquilizers causing CHD. A small increase in risk requires many more study subjects before the investigation has the power to demonstrate a difference between groups with a high level of certainty. Thus, a Type II error may have been committed. Even if there is no risk of tranquilizers causing CHD, this does not assure that there are not other adverse effects on the fetus that make tranquilizers unsafe for use during pregnancy. The investigators have therefore extrapolated beyond the data.

3. It is uncertain whether the difference in age between the two groups of women is related to their abortion status or their CHD status. If women are more likely to undergo induced abortion in their teenaged years rather than later in life, then this relationship alone may explain the differences in age between the groups. Even if the study had shown that the risk of CHD was smaller for teenaged pregnancies, the medical and social risks of teenaged pregnancy might outweigh this benefit. The mere presence of a statistically significant difference does not mean that a clinically important conclusion has been reached.

4. The difference between coffee drinkers and noncoffee drinkers is statistically significant but it is not large. A statistically significant result is one with a low probability of occurring by chance if there

are no true differences in the larger populations from which the sample data were drawn. However, it is clinically unlikely that such a small reduction in coffee consumption would have a large effect on the risk of CHD. Statistical significance must be distinguished from clinical importance and from contributory cause. Coffee drinking may have an effect, but with such small differences, one must be careful of attributing too much to coffee drinking.

5. By testing 100 variables, it is not surprising that the authors found associations that were statistically significant. The usual levels of statistical significance cannot be used to reject the null hypothesis of no association unless the relationship is hypothesized prior to the study. Thus, the authors cannot safely conclude that height and hair color are risk factors for CHD.

Exercise No. 2: Prospective Study

In an attempt to study the effects of a well-run cardiac care unit (CCU) on myocardial infarctions (MIs), investigators conducted a prospective study of the effects of a new CCU.

During the CCU's first year of operation, 40 patients were admitted to the CCU with diagnoses of "rule out myocardial infarction." Forty patients also were admitted directly to unmonitored wards with diagnoses of "rule out myocardial infarction." If cardiac enzymes were positive for MI in patients admitted to the CCU, lidocaine was started 24 hours after admission in an attempt to prevent arrhythmias.

In comparing the CCU patients with the ward patients, researchers found that the average age for CCU patients was 58 years versus 68 years for the ward patients. One-fourth of the CCU patients developed hypotension versus one-twentieth of the ward patients. Eighty percent of the CCU patients experienced ventricular arrhythmias versus 20% of the ward patients.

The researchers followed the patients during their hospitalization and for one year after hospitalization. They collected the following outcome data:

1. Thirty-six of the CCU patients eventually showed definite electrocardiogram or enzyme evidence of MIs versus 30 of the ward patients.

2. Eight CCU patients died in the hospital versus four ward patients. The differences were not statistically significant.
3. CCU patients remained in the hospital an average of 12 days versus 15 days for ward patients. The differences were statistically significant.
4. Among patients given lidocaine in the CCU, none died.
5. One year after discharge, former CCU patients were able to exercise an average of 20% longer than former ward patients.

The authors then drew the following conclusions:

1. CCU care causes a higher rate of development of MI among patients admitted to the hospital with chest pain.
2. Since the differences in death rates were not statistically significant, the authors concluded that CCU patients and ward patients had the same death rates.
3. Since the differences in length of hospitalization were statistically significant, the investigators concluded that they had demonstrated an important cost saving through use of CCU care.
4. Since lidocaine prevented all deaths if used after the definitive diagnosis of MI, the authors concluded that use of lidocaine upon admission to the CCU would eliminate all mortality due to MIs.
5. Since the CCU patients demonstrated greater exercise tolerance one year after discharge, the authors concluded that CCU care causes improvement in long-term survival.

Critique: Exercise No. 2
STUDY DESIGN
The investigators sought to study the effects of a well-run CCU unit, and chose to conduct their study in a new CCU. However, new facilities may not operate efficiently during the first year. Thus, the investigators may not have chosen an optimal setting for studying the effects of a well-run CCU. In addition the authors failed to state their specific hypotheses before conducting the study.

ASSIGNMENT
Selection bias may be present in this study if individuals with a poor prognosis were assigned to CCU care. This factor would be

important if physicians selectively admitted sicker patients to the CCU. There is some evidence that this was the case since a much higher proportion of CCU patients experienced hypotension. If physicians selectively admitted sicker patients with a poor prognosis to the CCU, then selection bias would be expected to affect the results of the study.

ASSESSMENT
The investigators found a much higher rate of arrhythmias among the CCU patients, which may have been the result of the method used for assessing arrhythmias. Since CCU patients were monitored continuously while those on unmonitored wards were not, it is possible that the intensity of observation of CCU patients uncovered a higher percentage of those arrhythmias that were present.

ANALYSIS
The researchers also found that CCU patients were younger, on the average, than ward patients. This factor may have occurred by chance or it may have resulted from the physicians' desire to provide more intensive care for younger patients. The age of patients is likely to be associated with certain outcomes such as exercise tolerance after MI. Thus, regardless of whether selection bias or noncomparability was responsible for age differences, age is a potential confounding variable which should be adjusted for in the analysis.

INTERPRETATION AND EXTRAPOLATION
1. The investigators found that a lower percentage of ward patients eventually showed evidence of an MI and concluded that the higher rate of MIs in CCU patients was caused by CCU care. The first requirement of establishing a cause and effect relationship is to establish that the cause precedes the effect. In this situation, it is likely that the patients already had experienced or were experiencing MIs when they were admitted to the hospital. Thus, in most cases, the effect (MI) may have preceded the cause (admission to the CCU). There is little evidence to support the interpretation that CCU care causes a higher rate of development of myocardial infarction.

2. The authors concluded that the death rates should be consid-

ered to be the same since no statistically significant difference in death rates occurred. The failure to demonstrate a statistically significant difference does not necessarily imply that no difference exists. When the numbers are small, it requires a very large difference to demonstrate statistical significance. The authors have not recognized the possibility of a Type II error. It is possible there were more seriously ill patients in the CCU group so that a higher death rate was probable than among the patients who were assigned to the wards. When the numbers are as small as the number of deaths in this study, it is better simply to state the number of deaths in each group without applying significance tests. In this study a difference did exist; even if the difference is not statistically significant, the number of deaths cannot be considered identical.

3. The CCU patients had a shorter length of hospitalization than the ward patients. The results were statistically significant, implying that the differences are not likely to be due to chance. Whether these differences are important from the cost standpoint is another question; the additional costs of CCU care may override the small differences in length of hospitalization. This consideration illustrates the distinction to be made between a statistically significant difference and an important difference.

4. Lidocaine was administered to CCU patients only after a definitive enzyme diagnosis was made and an MI was present at 24 hours. By this time the risk of death from an MI has greatly decreased, especially the arrhythmia risk. It is likely therefore that lidocaine administration had little to do with the fact that no deaths occurred among those given lidocaine. The authors have gone beyond the data in extrapolating their results to all CCU patients and did not recognize that the group of patients on lidocaine was different from patients newly admitted to a CCU.

5. The authors concluded that CCU care improved the prospect of recovery since CCU patients had a better exercise tolerance one year later. There is insufficient evidence to establish such a cause and effect relationship. Since CCU patients were younger than ward patients, they could be expected to have a better exercise tolerance. In addition, since more CCU patients died, there was a greater loss to follow-up in this group. The ability to survive an

MI may have selected out those with a higher exercise tolerance. Finally, there is no evidence presented that exercise tolerance one year after an MI is actually associated with improved, long-term survival. The authors should have been more careful about attributing a better prognosis to CCU care; in doing so, they extrapolated beyond the data.

Exercise No. 3: Experimental Study

A new vaccination for influenza was being tested. Participants were chosen for the study group by randomly selecting 1,000 families from a list of 5,000 who volunteered for the experimental trial. All 4,000 members of the families were given a vaccination. As a control group, the investigators randomly selected 4,000 individuals from the telephone directory and gave them placebo vaccination. In comparing the study and control groups, investigators found that the study group had an average age of 22 years versus an average age of 35 years for the control group. The study group was twice as likely to own a thermometer as the control group, but otherwise they were quite similar when compared on a long list of variables.

During the influenza season the following winter, each individual was instructed to see a study physician for any fever that occurred so that the possibility of influenza could be clinically evaluated. In their follow-up evaluation, the investigators gained the cooperation of 95% of the study group and 70% of the control group. They found that the control group had twice the attack rate of influenza as the study group and concluded that the new treatment cut the risk of influenza in half. The investigators recommended application of the new treatment to the general population in order to eliminate half the deaths due to influenza.

Critique: Exercise No. 3

STUDY DESIGN

The investigators failed to define what particular population they were using to try out the new therapy. It is not clear whether they were trying it out on families or individuals, on one age group or all age groups, on volunteers or the general population.

ASSIGNMENT

In experimental trials, investigators randomly and blindly assign volunteers to a control group and a study group. In this instance, all the volunteers were placed in the study group and given the experimental treatment. A separate population was then developed to produce the control group. Therefore random and blind assignment was not performed.

The investigators used different populations for selecting the study and control groups. To give all members of a family the new vaccine admits the possibility that a partially successful treatment will appear almost fully effective. If the risk to each family member is reduced slightly, the possibility of exposure within the family will be greatly reduced. Thus there are two factors that favor the vaccination: reduced exposure and increased immunity.

By selecting names from the telephone book, the investigators limited their control population to individuals listed in the telephone directory. This method did not result in a control population comparable to those receiving the treatment, particularly where children were concerned. Children are likely to be heavily represented in a population of families, but not in the telephone directory.

Even if a random sample of a population is performed, there is a possibility that the study and control groups will not have an equal distribution of attributes potentially related to a susceptibility to influenza. The age differences between the study and control groups (which might be expected from the method of assignment) need to be taken into account and adjusted for in the analysis. The difference in frequency of thermometer ownership, even if it occurred by chance, is an important difference since it could affect the recognition of fever. An increased recognition of fever is likely to result in an increased diagnosis of influenza.

ASSESSMENT

The method the investigators chose for assessment of influenza is not likely to be valid. Influenza is difficult to diagnose specifically and there are no standard criteria presented in the study for its diagnosis, such as culturing the virus. In addition, volunteers are likely to have a different threshold of illness before seeking medical care than nonvolunteers; this factor could have influenced the number of diagnoses of influenza made by physicians. Intensity of observation can differ between the groups, and this, too, may have affected the accuracy of assessment of outcome.

Finally, unless follow-up is complete, there is the possibility that those lost to follow-up actually had either a better or a worse outcome than those who can be traced. A large proportion of the control group in the study was lost to follow-up, which may have affected the validity of assessment of outcome. In general, the assessment of outcome in this study was not precise.

ANALYSIS

Since the populations differed in their age distribution, and age is a frequent factor influencing susceptibility, it is important to adjust the data for the effects of age. This could be accomplished by comparing the influenza attack rate of individuals of the same age to see if the differences between vaccinated and unvaccinated individuals remain the same. There was no statistical significance test applied to see whether the differences found were likely to be due to chance.

INTERPRETATION AND EXTRAPOLATION

The failure of this study to meet minimum standards for assignment, assessment, and analysis means that the study must be interpreted with great care. There are many explanations other than a causal relationship to explain the reduced number of diagnoses of influenza in the study group.

Extrapolation to other populations requires convincing proof of a causal relationship between factors in the study population; proof of a causal relationship was lacking in this study. Even if a relationship were established, one cannot extrapolate from influenza attack rates to death rates. The study, however, was not concerned with death rates and provided no evidence that the death rates were different in the two populations.

Controlled clinical trials (experimental studies) are the most powerful methods available for determining the effectiveness of medical intervention. But like retrospective and prospective studies, they must be thoroughly critiqued to prevent errors in assignment, assessment, analysis, interpretation, and extrapolation.

Review Exercise: A Prospective Study of Medical Screening in a Military Population

During their first year in the military service, 10,000 18-year-old privates were offered the opportunity to participate in a yearly health maintenance examination that included history, physical examination, and multiple laboratory tests. The first year 5,000 participated and 5,000 failed to participate; the 5,000 participants were selected as a study group, and the 5,000 nonparticipants were selected as a control group. The first-year participants were then offered yearly health maintenance examinations during each year of their military service.

Upon discharge from the military, each of the 5,000 study group members and each of the 5,000 control group members were given an extensive history, physical examination, and laboratory evaluation to determine whether the yearly health maintenance visits had made any difference in the health and life style of the participants.

The investigators obtained the following information:

1. On the basis of their reported consumption, participants had half the rate of alcoholism as nonparticipants.
2. Participants had twice as many diagnoses made for them during military service as nonparticipants.
3. Participants had advanced an average of twice as many ranks as nonparticipants.
4. There were no statistically significant differences between the groups in the rate of myocardial infarction.
5. There were no differences between the groups in the rate of development of testicular cancer or Hodgkin's disease, the two most common cancers in young men.

The authors then drew the following conclusions:

1. Yearly screening can reduce the rate of alcoholism in the military by one-half.
2. Since participants had twice the number of diagnoses made for them, their diseases were being diagnosed at an earlier stage in the disease process, at a point where therapy is more beneficial.
3. Since participants had twice the military advancement of nonparticipants, the screening program must have contributed to the quality of their work.
4. Since there was no difference in the rate of myocardial infarction, screening and intervention for coronary risk factors should

not be included in a future health maintenance screening program.
5. Since testicular cancer and Hodgkin's disease occurred with
equal frequency in both groups, future health maintenance examinations should not include efforts to diagnose these conditions.

Critique: Review Exercise

STUDY DESIGN

The investigators have stated only a general goal of studying the
value of the annual health maintenance examination. They do not
identify the population to which they wish to apply their results.
They do not state specific hypotheses or clearly identify their specific study questions.

If the investigators' goal was to study the effects of an annual
health maintenance examination, they have not accomplished this
goal since there is no evidence that first-year participants actually
took part in subsequent examinations.

Furthermore the authors' choice of study participants may not
have been appropriate for the study question. The study selected
young people who already had been screened for chronic illness
by virtue of passing the entry physical for military service. Being
a young and healthy group, they may not have been an appropriate
population for testing the usefulness of health maintenance for
older or high-risk populations in which the frequency of pathological conditions would be expected to be much higher.

ASSIGNMENT

Individuals in this study were self-selected, that is, they decided
whether or not to participate. The participants therefore can be
considered volunteers. There was no evidence presented by researchers to indicate that those who elected to participate differed
in any way from those who elected not to participate. It is likely
that participants had health habits and health risks that were different from those of the nonparticipants. These differences may
well have contributed to the difference in outcome. Since no baseline evaluation is available on the control group, it is not known
if or how they differed from the study group. Thus, one does not
know if the study group and the control group were comparable.

The individuals in both the study and control groups were self-assigned on the basis of their participation in the first year of the health maintenance examinations. Since the examinations were conducted on a yearly basis, those who initially participated may not have continued to participate. Thus, the study or control group status of the individuals involved may not have reflected validly their actual participation in the screening.

ASSESSMENT
Assessment of outcome was conducted only on those who were discharged from the military. Individuals who had died during military service would not have been included in those assessed at discharge. The individuals who died may have been the most important in terms of assessing the potential benefits gained by screening. This loss to follow-up may be a major error in the study.

Individuals participating in multiple health maintenance examinations were under much more intensive observation than the nonparticipants. This unequal intensity of observation may have resulted in a larger number of diagnoses being made for them during their military service. Nonparticipants may have had the same number of conditions, but not all of them resulted in a recorded diagnosis.

ANALYSIS, INTERPRETATION, AND EXTRAPOLATION
1. Participants had a lower rate of alcoholism than nonparticipants, perhaps as a result of differences between the groups prior to entry into the study. If heavy drinkers were less likely to participate in the health screening, then the screening would only seem to have altered the frequency of alcoholism. Comparative baseline data and adjustment for the differences was lacking in the analysis. In addition, the validity of the method used for assessment of alcohol consumption is questionable; since there were no uniform criteria for diagnosis, differences in recall and reporting were possible. Even if none of these potential errors existed, there is no evidence in the study that the screening, itself, was the causative factor in producing a lower rate of alcoholism. Extrapolating to the military in general was clearly beyond the range of the data.

2. The presence of more diagnoses of disease in the participants may merely reflect more intense observation because of more fre-

quent examinations. Many of their medical conditions may have been either self-limited or unaffected by current medical treatment. There were no measurements presented in the study indicating the stage of diagnosis of various conditions, and no data on the results of treatments. Thus, the benefits of early diagnosis and treatment cannot be made on the basis of this study.

3. If motivation is associated both with participation in the study and advancement in the military, then motivation would be a confounding variable, one related to both the attribute status and the outcome. Without controlling for this potentially confounding variable, no conclusion can be reached about the relationship between participation status and advancement.

4. Many of those with myocardial infarction may have died, and thus were excluded from the assessment. In addition, one would expect a very low rate of myocardial infarction in a young population. Even with the large numbers included in this study, the population may not have been big enough to demonstrate small differences between the groups. If one assumes that alterations in the risk factors that contribute to myocardial infarction also alter the prognosis, there is no indication here that those who participated had either more recognized risk factors or more risk factors altered. Even if they had more altered risk factors, the effects of these alterations may not become apparent until years after the participants have left the military. Therefore, this study was incapable of answering the question of whether screening for risk factors for coronary artery disease alters prognosis.

5. The absence of differences in the rate of development of testicular cancer and Hodgkin's disease cannot be assessed on the basis of those discharged alive. Even if the rates of development of the diseases were identical, it says little about the success or failure of the screening program. Success in screening for these cancers cannot be measured by the rate of development of the conditions since there is little known about methods for preventing these diseases. Thus, one would expect nearly identical rates of development of Hodgkin's and testicular carcinoma. The stage of illness at diagnosis and the prognosis for those who developed either of the conditions would be more appropriate measures for

assessing the success of the screening program. No such data are presented here, and thus, no interpretation can be made.

Having critiqued these flaw-catching exercises, the reader may feel discouraged; but, of course, most medical research studies have far fewer errors than the hypothetical exercises presented here. However, it may help the reader to remember that a certain number of errors are unavoidable and that detecting errors is not the same as invalidating research.

The practice of clinical medicine requires that clinicians act upon probabilities; therefore, a critical reading of the medical literature helps the clinician to more accurately define these probabilities. The art of reading the medical literature is the ability to draw useful conclusions from inconclusive data. Learning to detect errors not only helps the clinician to recognize the limitations of a particular study, but also helps to temper the unquestioned application of a study.

Testing a Test   PART 2

Introduction and Uniform Framework

Medical diagnosis may be regarded as an attempt to make adequate decisions using inadequate information. Thus the uncertainty that is inherent in medical diagnosis stems from the need to make diagnoses based on uncertain data. The diagnostic tools used in medicine have been regarded traditionally as a means of reducing the uncertainty in diagnosis. However, to successfully use diagnostic tests, one must appreciate not only how tests reduce uncertainty but also how they describe and quantitate the uncertainty that remains.

Historically, the diagnostic tools available were largely limited to a medical history and a physical examination. These are still powerful diagnostic tools. Today however, in addition to conventional methods, a massive array of ancillary technology, properly and selectively employed, can provide the thoughtful clinician with precise diagnoses. Learning if and when one should apply each element of the history, physical examination, and ancillary technology constitutes the essence of the practice of diagnostic medicine.

Today's emphasis on cost-conscious quality requires that physicians understand the fundamental principles of diagnostic tests: which questions they answer and which they do not, which tests increase the diagnostic precision and which merely increase the cost.

To paraphrase Will Rogers, physicians traditionally have believed that nothing is certain except biopsy and autopsy. However, even these gold standards for diagnosis may miss the mark or be performed too late to help. A knowledge of the principles of diagnostic tests helps to define the extent of diagnostic uncertainty as well as to increase certainty. Knowing how to live with uncertainty is a central feature of clinical judgment: the skilled physician has learned when to take risks to increase certainty and when to simply tolerate uncertainty.

The fundamental principle of diagnostic testing rests on the belief that individuals with disease are different from individuals without disease and that diagnostic tests can distinguish these two groups. Diagnostic testing, to be perfect, would require (1) that all individuals *without* the disease under study have one uniform value

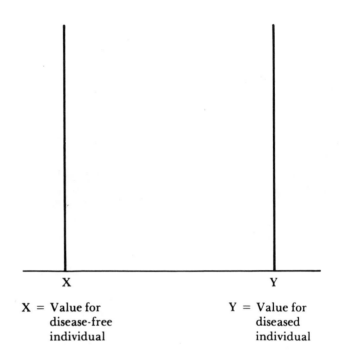

X = Value for
disease-free
individual

Y = Value for
diseased
individual

FIGURE 11-1. Conditions required for a perfect diagnostic test.

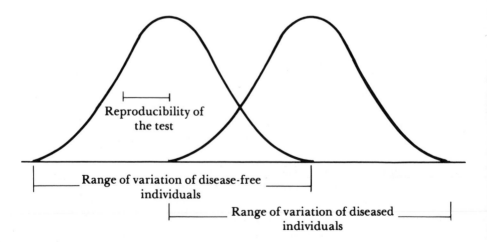

Reproducibility of
the test

Range of variation of disease-free
individuals

Range of variation of diseased
individuals

FIGURE 11-2. The three types of variations that affect diagnostic testing.

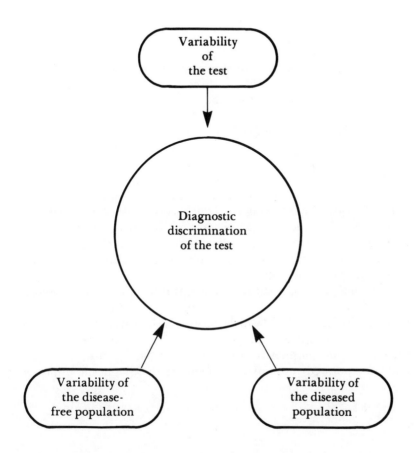

FIGURE 11-3. Uniform framework for testing a test.

on the test, (2) that all individuals *with* the disease under study have a different but uniform value for the test, and (3) that all test results be either those of the diseased or those of the disease-free group (Fig.11-1).

If this were the situation in the real world, then one perfect test could distinguish disease from health and the work of the physician would be merely to order the "right" test. The real world, for better or worse, is not so simple. None of these three conditions is usually present. Variations exist within each of the three basic factors: the test, the diseased population, and the disease-free population (Fig. 11-2).

The assessment of diagnostic tests is largely concerned with describing the variability of these three factors and thereby quantitating the conclusions that can be reached despite or because of this variability.

The variability, reproducibility, and accuracy of the test itself is discussed in Chapter 12. In Chapter 13 the variability of the disease-free population is reviewed and assessed using the concept of a range of normal. In Chapters 14 and 15 the variability of the diseased population and its relationship to the disease-free population is quantitated using the concepts of sensitivity, specificity, and predictive value. These concepts are outlined, and the errors in their implementation are illustrated. Flaw-catching exercises then provide an opportunity to apply these principles to the evaluation of diagnostic tests.

As with analyzing a study, it is helpful to have an overview, a generalized framework for evaluating a test. This framework is depicted in Figure 11-3, which illustrates the variability that exits in tests, in the disease-free population, and in the diseased population. It also emphasizes that these variations must be studied and incorporated into any assessment of the diagnostic utility of a test.

A perfect test would produce the same results every time it was conducted under the same conditions. In addition, its value would reflect precisely the true value that the test intended to measure. In other words, a perfect test would be completely reproducible and completely accurate. Let us first define these terms and see how they are used.

Reproducibility is the ability of a test to produce consistent results when independently performed and interpreted under the same conditions. Several factors, however, may affect the reproducibility of a test:

1. The conditions under which the test is reproduced may not be the same.
2. The repeat measurement may not be independent, that is, subsequent performance of the test may be influenced by the results of the first test.
3. The test may be affected by variations in interpretation from person to person. This effect is known as interobserver variability.
4. The test may be affected by variations in interpretation by the same person at different times. This effect is known as intraobserver variability.

In assessing the method for performance of the test, researchers must be sure that the technical and biological conditions for performance are identical when the test is repeated. Failure to follow this precaution results in the error illustrated in the following example.

The reproducibility of a test for serum cortisol levels was evaluated by drawing two samples from the same individuals. The first sample was drawn at 8:00 A.M. and the second at noon. Methods for performance were identical and interpretation was independent. This method was applied to 100 randomly selected individuals. The authors found that, on the average, there was a twofold difference between the serum cortisol levels found in the same individual. They concluded that the large variation indicated that the test was not reproducible.

Reproducibility is the ability of the test to produce nearly the same results when conducted under the same conditions. In this example, the investigators did not repeat the test under identical conditions. There is a natural cycle in the individual's cortisol level throughout the day. By drawing blood at 8:00 A.M. and again at noon, the investigators were sampling at two different times in the cycle. Even if this test were completely reproducible, the different conditions under which it was administered would produce quite different results.

Failure to perform truly independent measurements may allow the second reading to be influenced by the first reading as illustrated in the following example.

An investigator, studying the reproducibility of a urinalysis, asked an experienced laboratory technician to read a urinalysis sediment, leave the slide in place, and then repeat the reading in 5 minutes. The investigator found that the reading, performed under the same conditions, produced perfectly reproducible results.

In this example, the technician knew the results of the first test and was likely to have been influenced by the first reading when rereading the urine sample 5 minutes later. A measure of reproducibility requires independent measurements. Thus, the technician should not have known the results of the previous reading.

Even if interpreters are unaware of their own or other previous readings of the test, there is the possibility of individual variation. Whenever subjective judgment is involved in the interpretation of tests, there is room for inter- and intraobserver variations. Two radiologists frequently interpret the same X-rays differently; this is known as interobserver variation. An intern may interpret an electrocardiogram differently in the morning from his or her middle-of-the-night reading of the same test. This is known as intraobserver variation. These variations do not, in themselves, destroy the value of the test. They do require that the physician be alert to the constant probability of variation in interpretation. Inconsistencies of technique or interpretation contribute to some extent to a degree of variability in most tests. It is necessary therefore to have some criteria to judge how much variability can be tolerated.

In general, it is important that the variability of the test be much smaller than the range of variability due to biological factors. Thus the extent of variation in the test should be small compared to the range of normal for the test (see Chap. 13).

It is important to distinguish reproducibility from accuracy. The *accuracy* of a test is its ability to produce results that are close to the best available measure of the anatomic or physiological characteristic. The accuracy of a test is a measure of the precision of a test in comparison with other tests. A test may be very reproducible, yet quite inaccurate, reproducing results that are far from the true value. The following example illustrates a test of good reproducibility but poor accuracy, exemplifying the difference between reproducibility and accuracy.

A study was conducted on 100 patients undergoing surgery for navicular fractures. Each of the study patients had two independently interpreted X-rays, which were negative for navicular fracture within the week after their initial injury. The authors concluded that the radiologists had been negligent in missing these fractures.

Navicular fractures frequently are not diagnosed accurately by X-ray at the time of injury. Therefore, it may not be the negligence of the radiologists so much as the inaccuracy of the test that was used. Repeating the X-ray tests confirmed the reproducibility of the negative results by the radiologists. Accuracy, however, means that the test will produce a result that is close to the truth. Unfortunately, since X-rays are not always an accurate means of diagnosing navicular fractures, the test was at fault, not the radiologists.

A test may be quite accurate when employed in a scientific study, but it may lose its accuracy when applied in the "real world." It is helpful to think of two types of accuracy: (1) experimental accuracy—the precision of the test when applied under careful study conditions, and (2) field accuracy—the precision of the test when applied under real, clinical conditions. The difference between the two concepts is illustrated in the following example.

A study was conducted in a university hospital of 500 patients on a three-day, low-fat diet. It showed that the fat content in stools collected for 72 hours after the diet successfully separated those patients with malabsorption from those without it. An identical study protocol administered to 500 outpatients failed to identify successfully the presence of malabsorption. The authors of the outpatient study concluded that the inpatient results were incorrect.

The performance of a test is usually assessed under ideal experimental conditions. The field condition under which it is employed often may be less than ideal. A 72-hour stool collection after three days on a low-fat diet may be very difficult to collect on an outpatient basis. The fact that the outpatient data do not agree with the inpatient data may merely reflect the realities of the field conditions. While accuracy is a required property of a good test, the assessment of accuracy requires a comparison of the test with other more precise or more accepted measures; thus, it may not be possible initially to determine how accurate a test is. An assessment of the accuracy of a test may have to await the application of the test and its comparison with other diagnostic methods.

Disease-free human populations are subject to inherent biological variation. One need only to walk down the street to appreciate the differences between people. Individual height, weight, and color cover a span that reflects the wide, but not unlimited, variations that can occur among healthy individuals.

The concept of a range of normal is an effort to describe and quantify the range of values that exist among individuals believed to be disease-free. A range of normal can be derived from any measurement in which there are multiple possible values for disease-free individuals. These values would include physical exam characteristics such as blood pressure, liver size, and heart rate, or laboratory values such as hematocrit, sedimentation rate, or creatinine. Although the range of values is often wide, the concept does not include all those who are free of disease. It intentionally leaves out 5% of the individuals who are believed to be disease-free in order to create a range of normal that is wide enough to describe most disease-free values but not so wide as to include *all* possible values. The range of normal is *descriptive* not *diagnostic*. It describes disease-free individuals; it does not diagnose disease. Values outside the range of normal may be the result of chance variation, physiological changes unassociated with disease, or pathological changes secondary to disease.

Developing the Normal Range

The range of normal values is developed as follows:

1. The investigator locates a particular population of individuals who are believed to be disease-free. This population is known as the reference population. These individuals are frequently medical students, hospital employees or other easily accessible volunteers. They may be assumed merely to be disease-free or they may have undergone extensive tests and follow-up.

2. The investigator then performs a particular test on all the individuals within the reference population.

3. The investigator next plots the distribution of test values among this disease-free population.

4. The investigator then calculates a range of normal that includes the central 95% of the reference population. Some leeway is allowed in setting the upper and lower limits as long as the range of normal includes 95% of the reference group. Unless there is a reason to do otherwise, the investigator generally chooses the central part of the range so that 2½% of disease-free individuals have values above and 2½% of disease-free individuals have values below the normal range.

To illustrate the method for developing the normal range, imagine that investigators have measured the heights of 100 male students in a medical school and found values that looked like those in Figure 13-1. The investigators would then choose a range of normal that includes 95 of the 100 medical students. Unless they had a reason to do otherwise, they would use the middle part of the range so that the normal range for this population would be from 5 ft to 6 ft, 6 in. Individuals outside this range may not have any disease; they may be simply healthy individuals who are outside the range of normal.

Basic Principles

Let us look first at the implications of the concept of a range of normal and then illustrate the errors that can result from failure to understand these implications.

1. By definition, 5% of the population will have values that lie outside the range of normal on any particular test. Thus "abnormal" and "diseased" are by no means synonymous. The more tests that are performed, the more individuals there will be who are outside the range of normal on at least one test. Taking this proposition to its extreme conclusion, one might conclude that a normal person is anyone who has not been investigated sufficiently. Despite the absurdity of this proposition, it emphasizes the importance of understanding that the definition of the range of normal intentionally places 5% of a disease-free population outside the range of normal. Thus the term *outside normal limits* must not be equated with disease.

2. Values that lie within the range of normal do not assure that

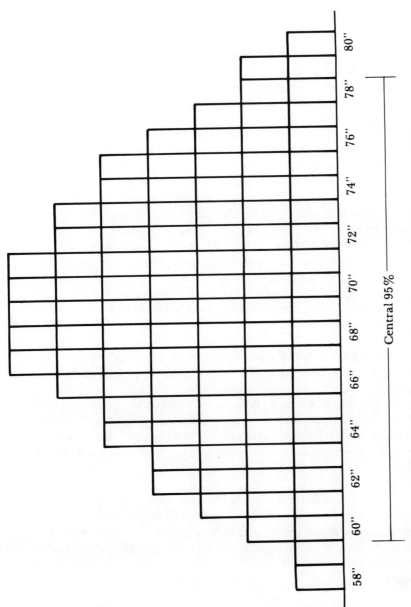

FIGURE 13-1. Heights of 100 male medical students used to derive a range of normal values.

the individual is disease-free. The ability of the normal range of the test to discriminate diseased from disease-free individuals varies from test to test. Unless the test is perfect in ruling out disease— and few tests are—some individuals with the disease will have values that lie within normal limits.

3. Changes within normal limits may be pathological. Since the range of normal includes a wide range of values, an individual's value may change considerably and still be within normal limits. For instance, the range of normal blood sugars may vary from 40 to 120 mg per 100 ml; the range of normal potassium may range from 3.5 to 5.4 mEq per L or the range of normal uric acid may range from 2.5 to 8 mg per 100 ml. It is important not only to consider whether an individual lies within normal limits, but also to consider whether the individual has changed over time. The concept of a normal range is most useful when no historical data are available for a comparison of individual patients. When previous results are available, however, they should be taken into account.

4. The range of normal is calculated using a particular population believed to be disease-free. Therefore, when applying a particular range of normal to an individual one must ascertain whether this individual has a reason to be different from the population used to calculate the normal range. For instance, if men are used to obtain a range of normal hematocrits, this range of normal cannot necessarily be applied to women who generally have lower hematocrits.

5. The range of normal must not be confused with desirable. The range of normal is an empirical measurement of the way things are among a population *currently* believed to be disease-free. It is possible that the entire population possesses values that are higher than ideal and may be predisposed to develop a disease in the future.

6. The upper and lower level limits of the range of normal can be altered for diagnostic purposes. The range of normal includes 95% of those who do not have a particular condition or disease. It does not require, however, that half of the individuals within

normal limits have values above the average and half of them below the average. There is some room for scientific judgment to determine where the upper and lower margins of the range of normal should be set. Where to set the limits depends on what a researcher or clinician desires to accomplish by using the test.

For instance, suppose that most of the individuals with a disease are found to have values nearer the upper limits of the range of normal for the test. If the investigator is willing to lower the upper limits of the range of normal, a larger proportion of those with the disease can be expected to have values above the range of normal. Then however, the investigator pays the penalty (or makes the trade-off) of labeling a larger proportion of the disease-free population as abnormal. At times it may be worth paying this penalty, especially when it is important to detect as many individuals as possible with the disease or when the follow-up testing to clarify the situation is cheap and convenient. This trade-off is illustrated in Figure 13-2.

By shifting the range of normal to the left as in the range of normal No. 2, note that area B becomes smaller than in the range of normal No. 1, and that area A becomes larger. In other words, a decrease in the number of false negatives leads to an increase in the number of false positives, and vice versa. More persons with the disease are now identified as outside normal limits by the test. At the same time, more individuals who are disease-free are classified as outside normal limits, therefore trading off more false positive readings for less false negative ones and vice versa. How many false positives and how many false negatives the physician or medical system is willing to tolerate, depends on ethical, economic, and political considerations as well as medical knowledge.

The following examples demonstrate errors that result from failure to apply each of these principles.

1. In a series of 1,000 consecutive health maintenance examinations, a series of 12 laboratory tests (SMA-12) was done on each patient even though no abnormalities were found on a medical history or physical examination. Five percent of the SMA-12s were outside the range of normal, a total of 600 abnormal tests. The authors concluded that these abnormalties fully justified doing SMA-12s on all health maintenance examinations.

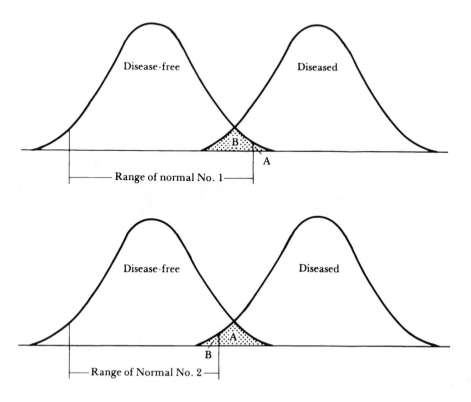

FIGURE 13-2. Shifting the range of normal. False positive, A: Individuals who are disease-free and who have values higher than the range of normal. False negative, B: Individuals who have disease and who have values within the range of normal.

Let us look at the meaning of these abnormal tests. A normal range of values, by definition, includes only 95% of those who are believed to be free of the condition. If a test is applied to 1,000 individuals who are free of the condition, 5% or 50 individuals will have values outside the range of normal. If 12 tests are applied to 1,000 individuals without evidence of pathology, then 5% of the 12,000 tests performed will be outside the range of normal. Five percent of 12,000 equals 600 tests. Thus, even if these 1,000 individuals were completely free of disease, one could expect 600 abnormal tests that merely reflect the method of determining the range of normal. Abnormal tests do not necessarily indicate pathology and do not by themselves justify doing multiple laboratory tests on all health maintenance examinations.

In considering the implications of an abnormal test, it is important to realize that all levels outside the range of normal do not carry the same meaning. Values well beyond the limit of normal may be considerably more important than values that are borderline. Values for outside the limits of normal carry a much greater likelihood of being associated with pathology whereas values nearer the limits of normal are more likely to be due to variation of the test or normal biological variation. For instance, if the upper limits of male hematocrits are 52 then a value of 60 is much more likely to be associated with disease than a value of 53.

2. One hundred chronic alcoholics underwent serum glutamic oxaloacetic transaminase (SGOT) determinations to assess liver function. The majority were found to have SGOTs within the range of normal. The authors concluded that these alcoholics had well-functioning livers.

This example illustrates the difference between range-of-normal laboratory tests and the disease-free state. The fact that these individuals had laboratory tests within normal limits did not establish that their livers were functioning properly since, on any one test, some diseased individuals will be within normal range. The poorer the capacity of the test to diagnose disease, the more individuals with disease will show values within the normal limits of the test. On certain tests diseased individuals may not be distinguishable from disease-free individuals. Both groups may have values in the normal range, which appears to have occurred in this study. The failure of the test to separate diseased from disease-free individuals indicates that the test had poor diagnostic discrimination and emphasizes the distinction between the range-of-normal limits and the disease-free.

Figures 13-3 to 13-5 illustrate three possible relationships between the disease-free and the diseased population. Figure 13-3 illustrates a test that completely separates those with disease from those who are disease-free. The diagnostic discrimination of this test is perfect. Figure 13-4 illustrates the usual situation in which

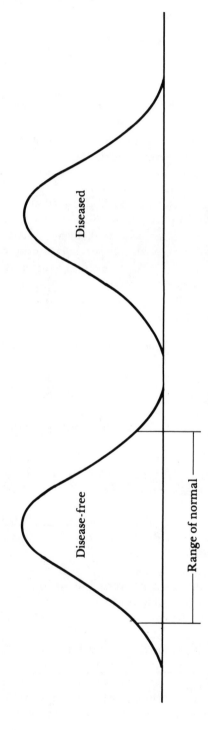

FIGURE 13-3. A test with complete separation of populations results in perfect diagnostic discrimination.

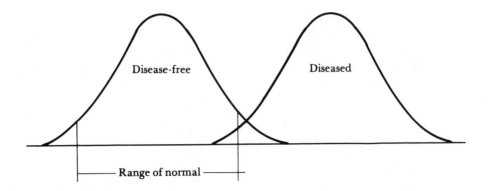

FIGURE 13-4. A test with partial separation of the populations results in partial diagnostic discrimination.

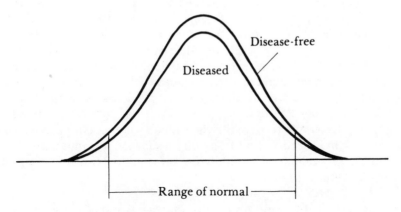

FIGURE 13-5. A test with no separation of the populations results in no diagnostic discrimination.

a test partially separates those with disease from those without disease. Figure 13-5 illustrates the situation in which a test has no diagnostic discrimination: individuals with disease have the same value as individuals without disease. In the SGOT example the situation closely resembles Figure 13-5. Despite its value in diagnosing many liver diseases, SGOT determination does not appear useful for diagnosing the chronic effects of alcohol on the liver. Thus despite the ability to calculate a range of normal for any test, the range alone will not indicate whether the test will be useful in diagnosis. Values for individuals with a particular disease may be identical with those of the disease-free population or vice versa, indicating that the test is of no value for diagnosing a particular disease.

3. Among 1,000 asymptomatic Americans with no known renal disease and with no abnormalties showing on urinalyses, normal values for serum creatinine were found to range from 0.7 to 1.4. A 70-year-old female was admitted to the hospital with a serum creatinine of 0.8 and was treated with gentamicin. Upon discharge, the woman was found to have a creatinine value of 1.3. Her physician concluded that since her creatinine was within normal limits upon admission as well as upon discharge, she could not have had renal damage secondary to gentamicin.

The presence of a value within the normal range does not assure the absence of pathology. Each individual has a disease-free value that may be higher or lower than the average value for the population. In this example, the patient increased her serum creatinine over 60% but still fell within the normal limits. The creatinine value prior to treatment suggests that its value after treatment was pathological, even if it was not outside the normal range for the population. It is possible that the gentamicin treatment caused renal damage, which was reflected in the woman's increased serum creatinine. When historical information is available, it is important to include it in evaluating a test. Changes within the range of normal *may* be a sign of disease.

4. A group of 100 medical students was used to establish the range of normal values for granulocyte counts. The range of normal was chosen so that 95 of the 100 granulocyte counts were included in the normal range. The range of normal granulocyte was determined to be 2,000 to 5,000. When asked about an elderly black male with a granulocyte count of 1,900, the authors concluded that this patient was clearly outside the values of the range of normal and needed to be further evaluated to identify the cause of the low graulocyte count.

The range of normal is dependent on the disease-free population chosen; it is usually defined as the range around an average value, which includes 95% of the individuals in a particular reference population who are believed to be disease-free. However, the disease-free reference population used for determining a range of normal values may have different values from the population to which one wants to apply the test.

It is unlikely that there are many elderly black males among the group of medical students used to establish the limits of normal. In fact, black males have a different range of normal granulocyte counts than white males. Thus, the range of normal established for the medical students may not have reflected the normal range applicable to the elderly black male, who was probably well within the normal limits for an individual of his age, race, and sex.

5. The normal range of serum cholesterol, as determined among 100 white American males aged 30 to 60, was found to be 200 to 300. A 45-year-old white American male was determined to have a serum cholesterol of 280. His doctor informed him that since his cholesterol was within normal limits he did not have to worry about the consequences of high cholesterol.

A normal value is calculated using data collected from a particular population currently believed to be disease-free. It is possible that the population used consists of many individuals whose values on the test are higher (or lower) than desirable. A normal value does not ensure that an individual will remain disease-free. It may be that American males as a group have higher than desirable cholesterol levels. If this is true, the patient with a cholesterol of 280 may well suffer the consequences of high cholesterol.

6. A study found that 10% of those with intraocular pressure greater than 25 mm Hg will develop visual defects secondary to glaucoma within the next 10 years. One percent of those with pressures between 20 and 25 mm Hg will develop similar changes, and .01% of individuals with pressures between 15 and 20 mm Hg will develop defects. The authors concluded that performance of the test could be improved by setting the upper limits of normal at 15 instead of 25 mm Hg since the test then could identify nearly everyone with the risk of developing visual defects (Fig. 13-6).

If 25 mm Hg is the upper limit of normal, then nearly everyone who will not develop glaucoma will be inside the range of normal, but a large number of individuals who will develop glaucoma will be included also within the normal range. On the other hand, if

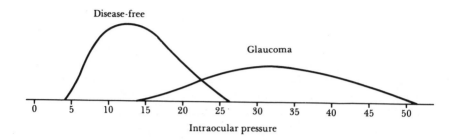

FIGURE 13-6. Possible distribution of intraocular pressure for those with glaucoma and those who are disease-free.

one sets the upper limits of normal at 15 mm Hg, very few individuals with glaucoma will be within the normal range, and a large number of individuals who will never develop glaucoma are outside the normal range.

The ability of a test to detect disease can be increased by altering the limits for the normal values. If the limits are extended far enough, the test will include nearly everyone with the condition. Unfortunately, this attractive solution also labels an increased number of individuals as abnormal who do not have nor will not have a pathological condition. By increasing the upper limits of normal, the investigators increase the ability to detect future disease, but only by paying the price of following up on a very large number of individuals who are destined to remain disease-free. In determining where to set the upper limits, the following factors might be considered.

1. Vision loss from glaucoma is largely irreversible and may develop before it is apparent to the patient.
2. Treatment is generally safe and effective in preventing progressive visual loss.
3. Follow-up is safe and involves little risk, or follow-up is time-consuming, requiring multiple, repeated examinations extending over long periods of time.
4. Follow-up produces anxiety among those for whom it is required.

The trade-offs then are not simply medical. Additional social, psychological, economic, and political considerations can all be incorporated into the decision of where to set the cut-off line. There may well be no correct answer. The only way out of this no-win situation may be to come up with a better test, one which has less overlap between those who will develop disease and those who will not.

The concept of a normal range is an attempt to deal with the variability that exists in the human population. An understanding of the utility and limitations of this concept is central to an understanding of diagnostic tests. The range of normal defines the values found for 95% of a particular reference population who are believed to be disease-free individuals, but they may not be desirable values, and they do not take into account changes from previous values.

The range of normal in and of itself tells us nothing about the diagnostic utility of a test. Every test has a range of normal that may or may not help in distinguishing individuals with disease from those without disease. To determine the utility of a test in diagnosing disease, it is necessary to look at the values of a population of individuals with a particular disease and to compare those values with the normal range of a disease-free population.

Having discussed and illustrated errors in assessing the variability of tests and the variability of the disease-free population, let us proceed to the variability of the diseased population.

Individuals with disease as well as disease-free individuals show a range of values on any test. The variability of individuals with disease may result from different severities of the disease or from differences in the individual's response to the disease. Despite this variability, it is essential to a study of the diagnostic discrimination of a test that a group of patients who have the disease under study be precisely and unequivocally defined.

The Gold Standard

The test or criterion used to define those who unequivocally have the disease is known as a *gold standard.* The gold standard may be a biopsy, an angiogram, a subsequent autopsy, or any other established test. The criterion of a gold standard in correctly identifying those with the disease is a necessary prerequisite to studying the diagnostic value of any new or unevaluated test; in other words, the value of the new test rests on its comparison with the gold standard. Thus a new test is compared to an older and better established test (or tests) to determine if it can do as well as the previous gold standard. Notice how it is assumed that, using the best of the older, established tests, it is possible to be 100% accurate—the assumption being that it is impossible to invent a better mouse trap since you can't do better than 100%. There might be a cheaper or more convenient mouse trap but, by definition, not one that is more accurate in catching its mouse.

It may sound like a "catch-22" to claim that the only way to evaluate a new test's diagnostic ability is to assume that it is already possible to make perfect diagnoses. Unfortunately, this is the position one is in when evaluating a new test. One only can ask whether the test measures up to the best of the old tests, that is, the gold standard.

Despite the inherent limitation of our ability to initially evaluate a new test, time and repeated application are on the side of the better mouse trap. Once applied in clinical practice, it may become evident that the new test actually predicts a subsequent clinical course better than the gold standard. It even is possible that eventually the new test will be accepted as the gold standard. Often, however, the problem is that definitive diagnosis is possible but is too dangerous or too late to be of maximum clinical benefit; in such instances, an adequate gold standard exists but not a clinically practical test. Under these circumstances, it is clinically beneficial to determine that a new test measures up to the gold standard. Once again one must understand that the goal of assessing a test is limited to comparing it with the best available test. Let us see what can happen when the gold standard is less than ideal.

One hundred individuals, admitted to a hospital with "diagnostic Q waves" on their electrocardiograms (ECG) and dying within one hour of admission, were autopsied for evidence of myocardial infarction (MI). Autopsy revealed evidence of MI in only 10. The authors concluded that the ECG was not an accurate method of making the diagnosis of an MI. They insisted on the gold standard of pathological diagnosis.

The accuracy of all diagnostic tests is determined by comparison to a gold standard test that has previously been shown to diagnostically measure the characteristic under study. Autopsy diagnoses are frequently used as a gold standard against which all other tests are judged. At times, even an autopsy is a less than perfect measure of disease, since the pathological criteria for MI may take considerable time to develop. It is possible that the diagnostic Q waves on an ECG are a more accurate reflection of an MI than pathological changes at autopsy. The investigator must provide evidence that the gold standard being used has in fact been shown to be the best available standard before using it as a basis for comparison.

Unfortunately, even the best available gold standards often do not unequivocally differentiate those with the disease from those without it. Investigators are often tempted to include only those who have clear-cut evidence of disease as measured by the gold standard. Despite the seemingly intellectual certainty that this provides, it may result only in a study of those with a severe or far advanced disease. This danger is illustrated in the next example.

In an effort to study the characteristics of individuals with hypertension, an investigator identified 100 individuals with diastolic blood pressure greater than 120 mm Hg. He found that all these patients had retinal vessel changes. He concluded that retinal vessel changes are essential to the diagnosis of high blood pressure.

It is difficult to know where to draw the line between hypertensive and nonhypertensive patients although it is generally agreed that diastolic blood pressures well below 120 are considered pathological. Many individuals with diastolic blood pressure in the hypertensive range— but below 120—may be free of retinal changes. Thus the investigator must be careful in using test criterion like retinal vessel changes that is primarily associated with severe or long-standing hypertension. As tempting as it is to study only individuals with clear-cut disease, it is deceptive to draw conclusions about all individuals with the condition only from a study of those with severe disease. In defining the diseased population, it is important to ask whether the best available gold standard was used to define the diseased population, and whether the diseased population spans the entire range of individuals who have the disease.

Even if these conditions are fulfilled, one must appreciate that the goal of testing a test is limited to determining whether the test being studied is as good as the established gold standard. The methods used do not address the possibility that the new test might be better than the gold standard.

CHAPTER 15

Diagnostic Discrimination
of Tests

It is now possible to derive measurements of the ability of a test to discriminate between those with disease and those who are disease-free. In doing so, it is important to remember the following three prerequisites for such an assessment.

1. Variability of the test: A measurement of the reproducibility of the test finding that the range of variability is relatively small in comparison to the range of normal
2. Variability of the disease-free population: A determination of the range of normal values for the test
3. Definition of the gold standard: Identification of groups of individuals who definitely have or do not have the disease

Sensitivity and Specificity

The traditional measures of the diagnostic value of a test are its sensitivity and specificity, which compare a test's diagnostic discrimination to a gold standard. Sensitivity and specificity have been chosen as measures because they are the inherent characteristics of a test that do not change when the test is applied either to a population where the disease is rare or to a population where the disease is frequent. They provide measurements of the diagnostic discrimination of a test that should be the same regardless of the population on which the test is used. *Sensitivity* measures the proportion of those with the disease who are correctly identified by the test. In other words, it measures how sensitive the test is in detecting the disease. *Specificity* measures the proportion of those who do not have the disease who are correctly called disease-free by the test.

Notice that sensitivity and specificity provide only the *proportion* of those with and those without a disease who are correctly categorized; these measures do not predict the actual number of individuals who will be correctly categorized. The actual number of individuals will depend on the frequency of the disease in the population being tested. Sensitivity and specificity are useful measures because they allow readers and researchers to compare test results performed on totally different populations. They evaluate the test, not the population on which the test is performed.

Let us first outline the mechanism for calculating sensitivity and specificity and then outline the implications and limitations. In calculating the sensitivity and specificity of a test in comparison to the gold standard, researchers proceed in the following manner.

1. The investigators choose the gold standard to be used in defining diseased individuals.

2. The investigators next choose one population that the gold standard indicates has the disease, and another population that—by the gold standard—does not have the disease. In implementing this criteria, it is important to know whether investigators included a representative group of individuals with and without the disease. In other words, do the individuals chosen represent a full spectrum of individuals who have the disease and who are disease-free, or do they represent only the two ends of the spectrum?

In choosing these individuals, it has become common practice to select as many diseased individuals as disease-free individuals defined by the gold standard. This 50–50 split, however, is not necessary since sensitivity and specificity are independent of the frequency of disease in the population being studied.

3. Researchers must now use the test being investigated to categorize all study individuals as positive or negative. In order to do this, they make use of the range of normal. If most individuals with the disease have values above the range of normal, then investigators use the upper end of the range of normal as the cut-off point between test positive and test negative. Conversely, the lower end of the range of normal is used if most values for those with the disease are below the range of normal. Using the cut-off point, investigators test all individuals with the new test and classify them positive or negative.

4. The investigators have now defined diseased and disease-free populations by the gold standard, and positive and negative by the test. They then can calculate the numbers of individuals for whom the test and the gold standard agree and the number of individuals for whom they disagree and display their results as follows.

TEST	GOLD STANDARD DISEASED	GOLD STANDARD DISEASE-FREE
Positive	a = Number of individuals diseased and positive	b = Number of individuals disease-free and positive
Negative	c = Number of individuals diseased and negative	d = Number of individuals disease-free and negative
	a + c = Total number of diseased individuals	b + d = Total number of disease-free individuals

5. Finally, investigators apply the definitions of sensitivity and specificity and calculate their values directly.

Sensitivity $= \dfrac{a}{a + c} =$ The proportion of the diseased labeled positive by the test

Specificity $= \dfrac{d}{b + d} =$ The proportion of the disease-free labeled negative by the test

To illustrate this procedure using numbers, let us imagine that a new test is performed on 500 individuals who are diseased by the gold standard and 500 individuals who are disease-free by the gold standard. We can now set up the 2 × 2 table as follows:

TEST	GOLD STANDARD DISEASED	GOLD STANDARD DISEASE-FREE
Positive	a	b
Negative	c	d
	500	500

Now suppose that 400 of the 500 diseased individuals are labeled positive by the test and that 450 of the 500 disease-free individuals are labeled negative by the test. One can now fill in the 2 × 2 table.

TEST	GOLD STANDARD DISEASED	GOLD STANDARD DISEASE-FREE
Positive	400	50
Negative	100	450
	500	500

Sensitivity and specificity can now be calculated.

$$\text{Sensitivity} = \frac{a}{a + c} = \frac{400}{500} = 80\%$$

$$\text{Specificity} = \frac{d}{b + d} = \frac{450}{500} = 90\%$$

Notice that the test has been applied to a population with 500 diseased and 500 disease-free individuals as defined by the gold standard. This 50% diseased and 50% disease-free population although arbitrary is the usual division chosen for study. The sensitivity and specificity would have been the same regardless of the number of diseased and disease-free patients chosen. One way to

convince oneself of the truth of this important principle is to look
at how the sensitivity and specificity are calculated, that is,

$$\text{Sensitivity} = \frac{a}{a + c} \text{ and Specificity} = \frac{d}{b + d}$$

Notice that a and c are both contained in the left-hand column of
the chart and that b and d are both contained in the right-hand
column of the chart. Thus the total number of individuals in each
column does not really matter since sensitivity and specificity relate
to the division of patients within a single column.

Having calculated the sensitivity and specificity, it is possible to
work backward and fill in the table when different numbers of
diseased and disease-free patients, as defined by the gold standard,
are used.

This time, however, let us assume that there are 900 disease-free
individuals and 100 diseased. These figures may approximate more
nearly the clinical situation in which the test is applied.

TEST	GOLD STANDARD DISEASED	GOLD STANDARD DISEASE-FREE
Positive	a	b
Negative	c	d
	100	900

Now let us apply the sensitivity and specificity measures as previously determined.

Sensitivity equals 80%; therefore, 80% of those with the disease
will be correctly labeled as positive (80% of 100 = 80). And 20%
of those with the disease will be incorrectly labeled as negative
(20% of 100 = 20).

Specificity equals 90%. Therefore, 90% of those who are disease-
free will be correctly labeled as negative (90% of 900 = 810). And
10% of those who are disease-free will be incorrectly labeled as
positive (10% of 900 = 90).

The following 2 × 2 table can now be constructed.

10% PREVALENCE

TEST	GOLD STANDARD DISEASED	GOLD STANDARD DISEASE-FREE
Positive	80	90 False positives
Negative	20 False negatives	810
	100	900

This is a situation where 10% of the population has the disease under study as the disease is defined by the gold standard so that the true prevalence of the disease is 10%.

Let us now compare this table to the one developed when sensitivity and specificity were first calculated. Since we used 500 diseased and 500 disease-free individuals, we were actually using a population with a 50% prevalence of the condition.

50% PREVALENCE

TEST	GOLD STANDARD DISEASED	GOLD STANDARD DISEASE-FREE
Positive	400	50 False positives
Negative	100 False negatives	450
	500	500

Notice that originally 100 individuals were falsely labeled negative and 50 were falsely labeled positive. In the population with 10% prevalence, however, 20 individuals were falsely labeled negative and 90 individuals were falsely labeled positive. The change in numbers is solely the result of the difference in prevalence in the two populations studied (50% versus 10%). Notice that in the 10% prevalence population, there are actually more positives who are disease-free (90) than positives who have the disease (80).

This fact may appear surprising in light of the high sensitivity and specificity; it is an important principle, however, that must be recognized in applying the concepts of sensitivity and specificity. Thus, despite the fact that sensitivity and specificity are not influenced by the prevalence of the disease, the actual number of individuals who are falsely labeled positive and falsely labeled negative is dependent on the prevalence of the disease. Let us illustrate the consequences of failing to understand and apply this principle with two hypothetical examples.

A test for liver disease with 80% sensitivity is applied to 1,000 members of a population with 1% prevalence of liver disease. Another test shown to have 95% sensitivity is applied to 1,000 members of a population with a 10% prevalence of liver disease. The authors conclude that since they are applying a more sensitive test to the population with 10% prevalence they can expect to have a smaller number of false negatives. The data from this study can be displayed as follows:

1% PREVALENCE

TEST	LIVER DISEASE	NO LIVER DISEASE
Positive	8	
Negative	2 False negatives	
	10	990

80% Sensitivity

10% PREVALENCE

TEST	LIVER DISEASE	NO LIVER DISEASE
Positive	95	
Negative	5 False negatives	
	100	900

95% Sensitivity

Sensitivity is a measure of the proportion of those with the condition who will be detected by the test. The actual number of individuals who will be missed, however, is also a function of the prevalence of the condition. Notice that despite the 95% sensitivity of the second test it produced five false negatives while the 80% sensitivity produced only two false negatives. Thus, fewer individuals would be missed when applying a test with 80% sensitivity to a population with 1% prevalence than when applying a test of 95% sensitivity to a population with 10% prevalence. The total number of individuals missed by a test is very much dependent on the prevalence of the condition.

Sensitivity alone therefore does not provide a good gauge of how many individuals will be missed by a test. The prevalence of the disease must be taken into consideration. In the same way, specificity is not enough to gauge how many individuals falsely will be labeled positive, as illustrated in the following example.

A test with 98% specificity is applied to 10,000 members of a population with 1% prevalence of the disease. The authors conclude that since the test is so specific, a positive test is diagnostic of the disease. This study can be diagrammed as follows:

$$\text{SPECIFICITY} = 98\% = \frac{d}{b + d} = \frac{9,702}{9,900}$$

1%
PREVALENCE

TEST	DISEASED	DISEASE-FREE
Positive		198 False positives
Negative		9,702
	100	9,900

Specificity is the proportion of those without the condition that the test correctly identified as negative. In this example, only 2% of those without the disease are incorrectly called positive by the test (false positives). This 2%, however, represents 198 individuals in this population. Since the condition is so rare, only 100 individuals actually have the disease; therefore the number of false positives is likely to be much greater than the number of individuals with the disease. Despite the high specificity of a test, a positive test may not indicate disease. In the case of a rare disease, even a very specific test may produce many false positives compared to the number of individuals who actually have the disease.

Predictive Value of Positive and Negative Tests

As previously discussed, the major advantage of sensitivity and specificity as measures of a test is their independence of the frequency or prevalence of the condition. This advantage is particularly useful for articles in the medical literature since it provides a measure of the value of tests that can be compared directly and used by others. Sensitivity and specificity, however, have shortcomings in answering two clinically important questions: If the test is positive, how likely is it that the individual is diseased? If the test is negative, how likely is it that the individual is disease-free? These are questions that are of practical concern to clinicians.

The measure that answers these queries is known as the *predictive value*.

Predictive value of a positive test = The proportion of those with a positive test who are diseased

Predictive value of a negative test = The proportion of those with a negative test who are disease-free

Unlike sensitivity and specificity, these measures answer the question of how good the test is at ruling in or ruling out the disease. The terms *prevalence* and *predictive value* are used in research articles dealing with groups of individuals. Fortunately, there are counterpart terms used in clinical practice where the clinician deals with one individual at a time. The *prevalence* of the condition means the same as the best estimate of the probablity of disease before performing the test. In clinical terms prevalence is known as *pretest*. The *predictive value* means the same as the probability of the disease being present or absent after obtaining the results of the test; this also is known clinically as *posttest probability*. If the terms *prevalence* and *predictive value* are confusing to you, substitute the concept of *probability of the disease* before and after the test.

Using 2 × 2 tables, let us illustrate how to calculate the predictive value. When calculating predictive value, remember to do so for one particular frequency or prevalence of the disease.

TEST	GOLD STANDARD DISEASED	GOLD STANDARD DISEASE-FREE	
Positive	a = Number of individuals diseased and positive	b = Number of individuals disease-free and positive	a + b = Total number of positives
Negative	c = Number of individuals diseased and negative	d = Number of individuals disease-free and negative	c + d = Total number of negatives

The following formulae are used for calculating the predictive value of a positive test and the predictive value of a negative test.

$$\text{Predictive value of a positive test} = \frac{a}{a+b} = \text{Proportion of those with a positive test who actually have the disease as measured by the gold standard}$$

$$\text{Predictive value of a negative test} = \frac{d}{c+d} = \text{Proportion of those with a negative test who actually are free of the disease as measured by the gold standard}$$

Let us now calculate the predictive values in the two populations we have already discussed. Remembering that the number of positives and negatives will be different for each prevalence of the disease, we can fill in the horizontal margins of the 2 × 2 table as follows:

	50% PREVALENCE POPULATION		
TEST	GOLD STANDARD DISEASED	GOLD STANDARD DISEASE-FREE	
Positive	400	50	450
Negative	100	450	550
	500	500	

	10% PREVALENCE POPULATION		
TEST	GOLD STANDARD DISEASED	GOLD STANDARD DISEASE-FREE	
Positive	80	90	170
Negative	20	810	830
	100	900	

The predictive values of both positive and negative tests are calculated as follows:

50% PREVALENCE

Predictive value of a positive test $= \dfrac{a}{a+b} = \dfrac{400}{450} = 89\%$

Predictive value of a negative test $= \dfrac{d}{c+d} = \dfrac{450}{550} = 82\%$

10% PREVALENCE

Predictive value of a positive test $= \dfrac{a}{a+b} = \dfrac{80}{170} = 47\%$

Predictive value of a negative test $= \dfrac{d}{c+d} = \dfrac{810}{830} = 98\%$

These calculations of predictive value have important clinical implications. They indicate that the probability of a disease being present or absent after obtaining the results of a test are dependent on the best possible estimate of the probability of disease made before performance of the test. When the probability of disease is moderately high before performance of the test—for example, 50%—even a negative test like the one used above leaves an 18% (100%–82%) chance that the disease is present. When the probability of disease is low before performance of the test, for instance 10%, even a positive test leaves a 53% (100%–47%) probability that the disease is absent. Failure to understand this concept can lead to the following error.

A new, inexpensive test for lung cancer is evaluated by applying it to a population of 100 individuals with lung cancer and 100 individuals with no evidence of cancer. A positive test is shown to have a predictive value of 85%, that is, 85% of those with a positive test have lung cancer. The authors conclude that this test is well suited for screening the general population since 85% of those with a positive test will have lung cancer.

The predictive value of a positive test is the percentage of those with a positive test who have the condition. The predictive value depends on the prevalence of the condition in the test population. In evaluating a test, it is often applied to individuals, half of whom are known to have the condition. In this example, the test was applied to a population in which 50% of the individuals had the condition (100 with lung cancer, 100 without lung cancer). Thus, the prevalence of the condition in the test population was 50%. The lower the prevalence of the condition, the lower the predictive value of a positive test. In the general population the prevalence of lung cancer will be much lower than 50%; therefore, the predictive value of a positive test when applied to the general population will be far below 85%. The ability of a positive test to predict disease is different in each population. A positive test may have a high predictive value in one population and be a very useful test; in another population, however, the same positive test may have a much lower predictive value. Such a test may be useful for diagnosis in a population with a high suspicion of disease, but it will be useless for screening a general population with low suspicion of disease.

A uniform framework for testing a test consists of an analysis of the variability of the test, the disease-free population, and the diseased population. This information is then combined with an assessment of the diagnostic discrimination of the test as measured by sensitivity, specificity, and predictive values.

The variability of a test is measured by its reproducibility, that is, independent repetitions of a test are performed and interpreted under the same conditions. Reproducibility does not in itself assure the accuracy or precision of a test. A reproducible test can reproduce imprecise results. Some variation is expected but it should be much smaller than the biological variation as measured by the range of normal.

Variability of the disease-free population is measured by the range of normal. By definition, the range of normal includes only 95% of those who are believed to be disease-free. The range of normal is dependent on the reference population chosen. Remember that the range of normal is merely descriptive of the way things are among a supposedly disease-free population. It is not diagnostic: Outside normal limits does not equal diseased; within normal limits does not equal disease-free; changes within the range of normal may be pathological; and within normal limits is not necessarily the same as desirable. The borderline for the range of normal may be adjusted to serve specific diagnostic purposes but the price paid in the number of false positives and false negatives must be taken into account. Finally, in using the concept of the range of normal to define a disease-free population, unequivocal limits must be set in order to determine which patients are positive and which patients are negative as measured by the test.

The diseased population is defined by the gold standard, which is generally accepted as the best test available for diagnosing the disease. In defining those with the disease, it is desirable to include individuals with as wide a range of pathology as possible.

Having determined that a test is reproducible, having defined both a positive and a negative test using the range of normal, and—using the gold standard—having identified a group of diseased and disease-free individuals, one is ready to assess the diagnostic discrimination of a test.

When the test under study is then applied to individuals who are identified as being diseased and disease-free, the sensitivity and specificity of the test is calculated *by comparing* the results of the test with the gold standard. Since the gold standard is assumed to have 100% or perfect diagnostic discrimination, the test under study will inevitably fall short of the gold standard; this is true even if the test is inherently better than the gold standard.

Sensitivity measures the proportion of those with the disease—as diagnosed by the gold standard—who are correctly identified as having the disease by the test under study. Specificity measures the proportion of those without the disease—as measured by the gold standard—who are correctly identified by the test as being disease-free. Sensitivity and specificity are important since they are independent of the prevalence of the disease in the population being studied and thus are inherent properties of the test. Different tests can then be compared to one another, using the measures of sensitivity and specificity.

Sensitivity and specificity, however, do not solve the clinical problem of what the probabilities are of the disease being either present or absent if the test is positive or negative. The predictive value both of a positive test and a negative test is necessary to determine how well the test rules in or rules out disease. The predictive value, unlike sensitivity and specificity, however, is dependent on the prevalence of the disease in a particular population. Clinically, this means that the clinician should make the best possible estimate of the probability of disease before performing the test. The predictive value then tells the clinician the probability of the disease being present or absent after performance of the test. The clinician should be careful not to extrapolate the predictive value from one clinical setting to another. A test that is very useful for diagnoses may be nearly useless for screening.

Laboratory Tests
Let us examine a few of the basic laboratory tests used in clinical medicine to assess their accuracy and reproducibility, range of normal, and diagnostic discrimination.

HEMATOCRIT
ACCURACY AND REPRODUCIBILITY. The hematocrit is a measurement of the percentage of the total blood composed of packed red

blood cells. Routine hematocrits are measured by either the finger stick method of assessing capillary blood or the venipuncture. Both methods can accurately measure the relative quantity of red cells, but reproducibility requires attention to technical detail. It must be noted, however, that capillary blood can be expected to have a hematocrit about 1%–3% lower than venous blood. Excessive squeezing of the finger tip can milk out extra plasma and falsely lower the hematocrit. When anemia is severe the finger stick measurement is less accurate.

In assessing the accuracy with which the hematocrit assesses the physiological status, remember that relative and not absolute red cell mass is being tested. Misleading results are possible when dehydration or diuresis lowers the plasma volume. Individuals with reduced plasma volume may present with hematocrits above the range of normal. These are normal variants but may be confused with polycythemia (pathologically elevated hematocrit).

RANGE OF NORMAL. Normal levels of the hematocrit are different for males and females. This is generally recognized and reported by laboratories as separate ranges of normal for males and females. Less often recognized are different levels of normal for different stages of pregnancy, different ages, persons living at different altitudes. The hematocrit normally falls during pregnancy beginning somewhere between the third to the fifth month. Between the fifth and eighth month, a reduction of 20% compared to previous levels is not unusual. The hematocrit generally rises slightly near term and should return to its previous level by six weeks postpartum.

Age has a pronounced effect on hematocrit, especially among children. The range of normal on the first day of life is 54 ± 10 (i.e., the range of normal is 44 to 64). By the fourteenth day the range is 42 ± 7. By six months the normal range is 35.5 ± 5. There is a gradual increase in the average hematocrit through the teenaged years, with the average reaching 39 between 11 and 15 years of age. Adult ranges of normal are for men 47 ± 5 and for women 42 ± 5.

Low barometric pressure has a pronounced effect on the range of normal hematocrits. Native residents who live at high altitudes have generally higher hematocrits. The range of normal at about 4,000 feet, for instance, is 49.5 ± 4.5 for adult males and 44.5 ± 4.5 for adult females.

The range of values for normal hematocrits is quite wide. Thus if an individual begins near the upper end of the normal range, as much as one-fifth of the red cell volume may be lost before anemia can be demonstrated by a low hematocrit. Comparisons with previous hematocrits are important in assessing the development of anemia. For any one individual the hematocrit is physiologically maintained within quite narrow limits.

DIAGNOSTIC DISCRIMINATION. When evaluating the hematocrit one must be aware of the method by which the hematocrit responds to acute bleeding. During the acute bleed, whole blood is lost and the remaining blood initially will approximate the original hematocrit. It may require 24 hours or more before compensation occurs through increase in the plasma volume and the hematocrit fully reflects the extent of blood loss. Failure to recognize this phenomenon leads to false negatives in recognizing acute bleeding.

The body is frequently able to compensate for slow blood loss or destruction. Therefore, despite an elevated reticulocyte count, patients with slow bleeding or hemolysis may not demonstrate anemia. If one expects to detect diseases predisposing to blood loss or destruction by ordering a hematocrit, then one will find a relatively large number of false negatives. Conditions like β-thalassemia and Glucose-6-phosphate dehydrogenase (G-6PD) deficiency often present as compensated anemia with a low normal or normal hematocrit. False positives may occur among those with expanded plasma volume as a normal variant. Looked at from another aspect, these individuals reflect the fact that for any range of normal some individuals without disease will have values outside the normal range.

BLOOD UREA NITROGEN (BUN) AND SERUM CREATININE

ACCURACY AND REPRODUCIBILITY. The BUN and serum creatinine are automated tests that are obtained quite reproducibly. BUN and serum creatinine reflect the serum accumulation of unexcreted urea nitrogen and creatinine, thus they reflect the inability of the kidney to excrete these substances. When used as measures of renal function, they attempt to assess the glomerular filtration rate. They are most accurate however in the presence of substantial renal impairment. The kidneys ordinarily possess considerable reserve function, thus substantial loss of function—one kidney for instance—may occur without increased accumulation of BUN and creatinine. Only after a 50% or greater loss of total glomerular filtration do the BUN and serum creatinine begin to accurately reflect glomerular filtration rate. As glomerular filtration rate decreases further, the BUN and creatinine start increasing at faster and faster rates. The percentage increase in BUN and creatinine rather than the numerical change more accurately reflects the percentage loss in glomerular filtration rate once BUN and serum creatinine are clearly elevated.

When the creatinine is within the normal limits and one needs a more accurate assessment of glomerular filtration rate, it is possible to get a twenty-four hour urine for creatinine plus a simultaneous serum creatinine, and to calculate the creatinine clearance. Although this test has its own problems with accuracy—reproducibility and range of normal—it is capable of detecting much smaller changes in glomerular filtration rate when the serum creatinine is not elevated.

RANGE OF NORMAL. The standard laboratory range of normal for BUN is 10–20 mg/dl and for creatinine 0.6–1.4 mg/dl. Utilizing these ranges of normal requires an understanding of the factors that affect these levels in the absence of disease. BUN is a reflection of the protein status and hydration of a patient. Thus a patient's values can change substantially without indicating specific disease. Creatinine is a product of muscle and, as such, varies widely among disease-free individuals according to their muscle mass. Women generally have lower creatinine levels than men and the elderly as a group have lower muscle mass and comparable lower serum creatinines. Despite these substantial differences, laboratories generally report creatinine levels as a single range of normal.

Creatinine as opposed to BUN varies less from day to day and month to month in response to non-renal factors. Comparisons of creatinine with previous levels can often provide important information about renal status. A serum creatinine level of 1.3 for an elderly female may reflect considerable loss of glomerular filtration rate especially if it has increased compared to previous determinations. The same level for a muscular young man may be stable and will give no indication of diminished glomerular filtration rate.

DIAGNOSTIC DISCRIMINATION. False negatives for renal disease using the BUN and creatinine are very common since, as previously discussed, BUN and creatinine do not begin to rise until substantial loss of glomerular filtration has occurred. In addition, false positives occur with both BUN and creatinine. BUN levels may be low in diseases that lead to malnutrition. Alcoholics, for instance, frequently have low BUN levels. BUN also reflects blood breakdown that occurs during rapid loss of blood into the GI tract. These elevations of BUN are not strictly false positives since they indicate diseases other than renal diseases. They are false positives, however, if one is trying to assess glomerular filtration. Falsely elevated creatinine can occur in the presence of muscle disease. Again, these are not really false positives, but they suggest a disease other than renal disease.

It is possible to use the BUN and creatinine together to help understand and localize the abnormalities. Ordinarily the ratio of BUN to creatinine is about 15:1. Elevations of BUN out of proportion to creatinine is suggestive of pre- or postrenal disease rather than intrinsic kidney disease. Thus dehydration generally will give a prerenal pattern of BUN elevated out of proportion to creatinine. Occasionally, one will find a postrenal disease such as prostate obstruction that also results in a BUN elevated out of proportion to creatinine.

URIC ACID

ACCURACY AND REPRODUCIBILITY. Uric acid levels in the blood can be measured reproducibly using automated techniques. There are several different methods, each of which gives slightly different levels. It is important to compare values obtained by the same method. Automated techniques generally give slightly higher values. Levels of uric acid can vary over short periods of time. Dehydration, for instance, can rapidly and significantly increase uric acid.

Uric acid blood levels accurately measure the uric acid in the serum. They do not, however, accurately assess all the important physiological parameters of uric acid. They are not an accurate gauge of total body uric acid. Crystalized and deposited uric acid, for instance, is not included in the serum measurement. With respect to the development of gout, crystalized and deposited uric acid is often the governing consideration. In addition, uric acid serum levels are only one factor affecting the excretion of uric acid. Some individuals without a high level of serum uric acid may excrete large quantities of uric acid predisposing them to uric acid stones.

RANGE OF NORMAL AND DIAGNOSTIC DISCRIMINATION. The range

of normal values for uric acid is quite wide, with the range of normal varying from about 2 mg/dl to 8 mg/dl in most laboratories with some variation depending on the method used. A large number of individuals are found with values slightly above this range of normal and very few below this range. Very few individuals with values only slightly above this range develop gout. This has caused many physicians to argue that slightly high levels of uric acid should not be treated. They are really arguing that the upper range of normal should be increased so that the serum level of uric acid can better discriminate those who are predisposed to gout from those who are not.

Even at high levels of uric acid, the diagnostic discrimination is not perfect. False positives occur frequently. Individuals with renal failure often have very high serum uric acid but rarely develop gout. Obviously, there are other factors besides serum uric acid level that determine the development of gout. In predisposed individuals, gout has been shown to develop at times when the uric acid blood levels were changing rapidly. Reductions as well as increases can precipitate gout. Individuals with gout not infrequently have uric acid serum levels within the range of normal when they present with gout. These cases are documented by demonstration of birefringent crystals in the joint fluids and not by their serum level of uric acids. Those suspected of gout, but with levels of uric acid within normal limits during their acute attack, should be rechecked at a later time. Their uric acid levels then will often be increased, demonstrating the existence of a false negative at the time of onset of gout.

Because of the poor correlation of serum uric acid and urine excretion, serum uric acid can be said to have poor diagnostic discrimination for uric acid stones. The number of false positives and false negatives would be very large if one used serum levels as a major diagnostic criterion. Actual demonstration of uric acid stones is the most definitive method of diagnosis. Twenty-four-hour urine excretion of uric acid is also an important method. Markedly increased 24-hour uric acid urine excretion has been shown to predispose to uric acid stones. The correlation here, however, is not one-to-one either, since many other factors affect stone formation. A low urine volume and a low urine PH, in particular, are important predisposing factors increasing the frequency of uric acid stones.

Uric acid demonstrates several important principles applicable to diagnostic tests.

1. Even in the presence of an accurate and reproducible test that reflects the metabolic abnormality linked to disease, there may be a poor correlation of serum level and the existence of pathology.
2. Serum levels as measured in uric acid and many other tests may not be a good reflection of total body levels, in particular, levels at the site of the pathology.
3. Serum levels may be least dependable at the time when they are needed most, at the time of onset of symptoms.

Questions to Ask in Testing a Test

The following checklist of questions to ask should help to reinforce the principles involved in testing a test.

1. Inherent Properties of a Test
   a. Independent reproducibility: Do multiple independent repetitions of the test under the same conditions produce nearly identical results?
   b. Technical reproducibility: Are there technical factors in the performance of the test that lead to inconsistent results?
   c. Independence: Were the results of the repetition obtained without knowledge of the initial results?
   d. Interobserver variability: Are there important variations between interpreters of the test that produce interobserver variability?
   e. Intraobserver variability: Are there variations between results obtained by the same interpreter repeating the test?
   f. Accuracy: Has the accuracy of the test been distinguished from the reproducibility of the test?
   g. Experimental accuracy: Under experimental conditions, has the test been shown to produce values that are close to the best available measure of the true value?
   h. Clinical accuracy: Under conditions of actual clinical performance has the test been shown to produce values that are close to the experimentally derived value?

2. Biological Variation: The Concept of the Range of Normal and Variability of the Disease-free Population
   a. Has a range of normal been properly obtained to include 95% of those believed to be free of disease?
   b. Has the disease-free reference population chosen been compared to other reference populations to determine whether the normal range being used is generally applicable?
   c. If the range of normal is not generally applicable, are different ranges of normal available for different reference populations?
   d. Have investigators recognized that values outside normal limits by definition include individuals who are disease-free?
   e. Have those who apply the test recognized that the range of normal is a description of a population and that changes within the normal range for any one individual may be pathological?
   f. Have the advocates of the test distinguished the range of normal from desirable?
   g. Have the investigators defined the range of normal as a symmetrical distribution above and below the average value or have they justified moving the range of normal to accomplish specific diagnostic goals?
3. Variability of the Diseased Population
   a. Have the investigators chosen the best available gold standard for defining which patients have the disease under study?
   b. Have the investigators included a broad enough cross-section of those with the disease to produce a realistic range of values for those with the disease?
4. Diagnostic Discrimination: Distinguishing Diseased from Disease-free Individuals
   a. In comparing the diseased and disease-free populations, how well does the test identify those with disease? How high is its *sensitivity* in detecting disease?
   b. In comparing diseased and disease-free individuals, how well does the test identify those who are disease-free? How high is its *specificity* in identifying disease-free individuals?
   c. Have the advocates of the test recognized that specificity and sensitivity alone do not allow one to predict the probability of disease from a negative or a positive test?

d. Have the advocates of the test recognized the extreme importance of the prevalence of the disease in obtaining a *predictive value* of disease from a positive or a negative test?

The following exercises are designed to evaluate your ability to apply the various principles used in testing a test. The exercises include a variety of errors, which have been illustrated in the hypothetical examples. Read each exercise, then write a critique pointing out the types of errors committed by the investigators. Compare your critique to the sample critique provided.

Exercise No. 1: Variability of the Diseased and the Disease-free Populations

Two investigations were conducted to evaluate the diagnostic value of a new test for breast cancer. The test had previously been shown to have values that varied by less than 1% when repeated under the same conditions by the same interpreter.

In the first study, the investigators chose 100 women with metastatic breast cancer and 100 healthy women without any signs of breast disease. Values on the test for the healthy women were 30 to 100. Values for breast cancer patients ranged from 150 to 200. Since this test perfectly separated the populations, the investigators concluded that it could be considered an ideal test for diagnosing breast cancer and should immediately be applied to screening the general population.

In a second study using the same test, another investigator compared 100 newly diagnosed breast cancer patients to 100 patients with benign breast disease. The cancer patients' values ranged from 70 to 200 while the patients with benign breast disease ranged from 40 to 180. The authors of this study noted the tremendous overlap between the two groups and concluded that the test was worthless.

A reader of these studies could not understand how two respected investigators could produce such inconsistent results. He concluded that there must have been errors in reporting the test values.

Critique: Exercise No. 1

To review these studies, it is helpful to organize the discussion by using the concepts of the variability of the test, the variability of the disease-free population, and the variability of the diseased population.

VARIABILITY OF THE TEST

Reproducibility is the measure of the variability of the test. The study states that the test had previously been shown to have had only a 1% variation when conducted under the same conditions by the same interpreter. A measure of reproducibility also requires independent performance of the test so that the second performance is not influenced by the results of the first test. The same interpreter performed the repetition of the test results, thus it is possible that he or she was influenced by the initial values. If this were true, then the reproducibility using independent interpretations might be far less than was previously reported. In the rest of this discussion, however, let us assume that the authors are correct in believing that the test is reproducible.

VARIABILITY OF THE DISEASE-FREE POPULATION

The first study used healthy patients and found a range of values from 30 to 100. In contrast, the second study used women with benign breast disease and found values of 70 to 200. These two studies may not be in contradiction; they may represent two different segments of the breast cancer-free population. It is possible that benign breast disease raises the levels of the test to intermediate values.

The proper measure of the disease-free population is the range of normal, which includes 95% of the breast cancer-free population. Results here, however, are presented as ranges that include 100% of the individuals; the total range tells nothing about how the values are concentrated. The values may be concentrated heavily between 70 and 100. Without all the data or at least a range of normal, it is difficult to use these studies to compare patients without breast cancer to patients with breast cancer.

VARIABILITY OF THE DISEASED POPULATION

The first study used patients with metastatic breast cancer and found a range of values from 150 to 200. The second study used newly diagnosed breast cancer patients and found a range from 70 to 200. This discrepancy may not reflect error in reporting the data; it may reflect the different populations used. Newly diagnosed breast cancer patients are likely to reflect a wide spectrum of those with the disease. Individuals with early disease as well as metastatic disease are likely to be represented among newly diagnosed patients. Metastatic breast cancer patients, however, may reflect only one end of the spectrum of disease. Thus, the wider range of values found among the newly diagnosed patients may reflect the more representative breast cancer population used in the second study.

DIAGNOSTIC DISCRIMINATION

The data presented does not allow one to calculate the sensitivity or specificity of the test. There is no mention of the distribution of individual values so it is not possible to obtain a range of normal or a division between positive and negative tests. Therefore, no conclusions are warranted about the diagnostic utility of the test.

In the first study, the investigators used individuals with a far-advanced disease and individuals who were clearly disease-free. It is not surprising that their test results appeared to separate the populations successfully. In the second study, the investigators included a wider spectrum of the diseased and also included those with benign breast disease. Therefore it also is not surprising that there was more overlap of values in this second study. The interpretation of the first study as a perfect test and the second study as a worthless test are both incorrect. The truth, which probably lies somewhere in between, requires an assessment of sensitivity and specificity using all the data from a wide spectrum of the diseased and the disease-free populations.

Exercise No. 2: The Concept of Normal

An investigator attempts to derive the limits of normal for a new test for diabetes in the following way.

1. He locates 1,000 hospital patients admitted for primary conditions other than diabetes.
2. He performs the new test on all 1,000 patients.
3. He plots out the values for the new test, excludes the top 2½% and the bottom 2½%, and includes the other 95% as the normal range.

The investigator now takes his new test to the community and performs screening tests on all volunteers. He tells all those who fall within the normal range that they are free of diabetes and tells all those who fall outside the normal range that they have diabetes. One year later he goes back to several individuals whose values fell at the low end of the normal range and retests them. He finds that they are now at the upper end of the normal range and he assures them that they are free of diabetes.

An obese male patient with values at the high end of normal and a strong family history of diabetes asks for advice on how to avoid developing the disease. The investigator advises him that since he is within the normal range he has nothing to worry about.

Critique: Exercise No. 2
DEVELOPMENT OF THE RANGE OF NORMAL

In developing the normal range, an investigator should seek to include only individuals who are free of the disease under study. The investigator in the above study concluded that individuals admitted with diagnoses other than diabetes were free of diabetes. Diabetes, however, is a very common condition and diabetics develop a series of complications that increase their risk of being hospitalized. Therefore it is likely that a proportion of individuals admitted with other primary diagnoses also had diabetes. The investigator may not have developed his range of normal from diabetes-free patients.

The investigator used the central 95% of the population's values as the range of normal. This is the usual procedure, but it may not maximize the diagnostic discrimination of the test. By altering the limits of the range of normal, it is sometimes possible to improve the ability of the test to discriminate between those with and those without the disease. It must be remembered, however, that when one changes the limits of the range of normal, one then pays the penalty of labeling more disease-free individuals as abnormal. This penalty however may be worth the price, but further data are required before one can know this. In any event, these data do not provide adequate means of judging whether this new test helps to discriminate between diabetics and nondiabetics. There was no external gold standard used to define who actually had diabetes. All we know is the range of normal for the test.

APPLYING THE RANGE OF NORMAL

The distinction between the concept of the range of normal and the concept of pathology has not been maintained. The author has equated *outside the range of normal* with diabetes and *within the range of normal* as free of diabetes. There is no evidence presented that the new test is of any value in discriminating diabetics from non-diabetics. It is possible that diabetics fall entirely within the normal range on this test.

Even if this test had been shown to be of value in separating those with diabetes from those without diabetes, there still would exist a few individuals with diabetes within the normal range as well as diabetes-free individuals outside the normal range. By definition, the normal range excludes 5% of individuals who are free of the disease. Thus the investigators cannot simply apply the test and label individuals as diabetics or nondiabetics.

CHANGES WITHIN THE RANGE OF NORMAL
When an individual changes values within the normal range, however, it could be a manifestation of pathology. The concept of the normal range is developed primarily for individuals for whom no previous baseline data is available. When this is the case, it is necessary to compare an individual's current values to those of supposedly disease-free individuals using the established range of normal. If the same test has been run on the individual previously, this information should be taken into account.

A change within the normal range may represent a large increase for a given individual; this is especially true if a patient previously had been near the lower limits of the range of normal and then moved to the upper limits. For these individuals, changes within the normal limits may be early manifestations of disease.

REFERENCE POPULATION
The reference population used in the study to develop the range of normal were all hospitalized patients. Their range of normal may have been quite different from those of a younger, ambulatory, and otherwise healthy population. Thus, an error may have been introduced by developing the limits of normal from one population and applying it to another population with different characteristics.

NORMAL VERSUS DESIRABLE
It is possible that all or some of those individuals whose values on the test are within normal limits have values that are higher than

desirable. Remember that the normal range is a reflection of the way things are, not necessarily of how they should be ideally. It is possible that losing weight and thus lowering the values of the test will prevent future problems. Of course this assumes that the test in fact discriminates between diseased and nondiseased, that losing weight will affect the test levels, and that lowered test levels carry a better prognosis. The general point, however, is that values within the normal range are not necessarily desirable values.

Exercise No 3: Diagnostic Discrimination of Tests

The usefulness of a new test for thrombophlebitis is being tested. The traditional gold standard for thrombophlebitis has been the venogram to which the new test is being compared. To assess the reproducibility of the new test, it is performed on 100 consecutive patients with positive venograms. The investigators find that 95% of the patients diagnosed as having thrombophlebitis record a positive value. The investigators now repeat the test on the same group of patients. They again find that it is positive in 95% of the 100 patients. From this they conclude that the new test is 100% reproducible.

Having demonstrated the reproducibility of the new test, the authors proceed to study its diagnostic discrimination. The authors evaluate the success of the new test as measured against the venogram, the traditional gold standard. They study 1,000 consecutive patients with unilateral leg pain, 500 of whom have positive venograms and 500 of whom have negative venograms. Having previously defined the limits of normal on the new test, the investigators classify individuals as positive or negative and present their data as follows.

NEW TEST	POSITIVE VENOGRAM	NEGATIVE VENOGRAM
Positive	450	100
Negative	50	400
	500	500

The investigators use the accepted definition of sensitivity, that is, sensitivity is the proportion of those with a positive test by the gold standard who have a positive test using the new test. Thus,

$$\text{Sensitivity} = \frac{450}{500} = 90\%$$

They use the accepted definition of specificity, that is, specificity is the proportion of those with a negative test by the gold standard who have a negative test using the new test. Thus,

$$\text{Specificity} = \frac{400}{500} = 80\%$$

They calculate the predictive value of a positive test for their study population. The accepted definition of the predictive value of a positive test is the proportion of those with a positive new test who actually have the condition as measured by the gold standard. Thus,

$$\text{Predictive value of a positive test} = \frac{450}{550} = 81.8\%$$

From these results, the investigators are led to the following conclusions.

1. The new test is completely reproducible.
2. The new test is less sensitive and less specific than the venogram thus it is an inherently inferior test.
3. When applied to a new population—for instance, a population with bilateral leg pain—a positive new test can be expected to have a predictive value of 81.8%. For individuals with bilateral leg pain and a positive new test, 81.8% would have a positive venogram indicative of thrombophlebitis.

Critique: Exercise No. 3
If a test is performed several times on the same individuals under the same conditions, the method of assessing reproducibility requires that the results for each individual be nearly identical. The

authors state that the total number of positive new tests was identical when the test was repeated. They do not, however, indicate whether the same individuals were positive upon repetition of the test as were positive the first time the test was performed. If the same individuals were not positive, the test could not be considered highly reproducible. The authors also fail to indicate whether those who performed and interpreted the repetition of the test knew of the results of the first test, and therefore the independence of the measurements cannot be assessed.

A gold standard is a generally accepted measure of a disease against which new or unproven measures are compared. The gold standard traditionally used may not be in fact a completely accurate measure of the disease it is designed to measure. A test is used as a gold standard only because tradition or general acceptance have established its usefulness. It is possible however for a new test to be a more accurate measure of the disease than the accepted gold standard. When comparing the sensitivity and specificity of new tests to that of the gold standard, it must be kept in mind that disagreement between the tests may result from the inaccuracy of the gold standard instead of the inaccuracy of the new test. This inherent limitation of the method for measuring diagnostic discrimination must be kept in mind.

When the authors conclude that the new test is less specific and sensitive than the venogram, they are assuming that the venogram is 100% sensitive and 100% specific. When one makes this assumption there is no way for the new test to be more specific or more sensitive than the old test. Unless one can be sure of the complete accuracy of the venogram, it is premature to conclude that the new test is a less useful measure of thombophlebitis. The authors therefore should limit their conclusions about the sensitivity and specificity of the new test to a comparison with the venogram.

The authors have correctly measured the sensitivity, specificity, and predictive value of their study population. As they state the predictive value of a test is the proportion of those with a positive new test who actually have the condition as measured by the gold standard. In this study population the prevalence of thrombophlebitis is 50% (500 with thrombophlebitis, 500 without) and the predictive value of the test is 450/550 equals 81.8%. The predictive value of a test however is different in each population, depending on the prevalence of the condition in the population. One cannot extrapolate a predictive value derived in one population directly to another population with a different prevalence of the condition. One would expect that patients with unilateral leg pain would have a different prevalence of thrombophlebitis from a population with bilateral leg pain. If one can estimate the percentage of those with bilateral leg pain who have thrombophlebitis, then it is possible to calculate the predictive value of a positive test in patients with bilateral leg pain. Let us assume that the prevalence of thrombophlebitis is much lower among patients with bilateral leg pain. One would then expect that a positive new test would have a much lower predictive value than for a population with unilateral leg pain.

Remember that, clinically, the prevalence is the same as the probability of the disease being present before the test is performed, and the predictive value of a positive test is the probability of the disease being present after obtaining a positive test. Since the probability of thrombophlebitis in a patient who presents with bilateral leg pain is much lower than 50%, the probability of disease even after a positive test would be far below 81.8%.

Rating a Rate

PART 3

Introduction and Uniform Framework

When you hear hoof beats, it is more likely to be a horse than a zebra. This clinical pearl stresses the obvious but too often forgotten truth that common diseases occur commonly and rare diseases occur rarely. When clinicians say that one disease is common and another is rare, they are implying a difference in rates.

All clinicians instinctively use a concept of rates. They know that coronary artery disease is much more likely in a middle-aged man than in a teenaged woman. They know that pancreatic cancer is much more common in an elderly person than in a young person. They know that sickle-cell anemia is much more likely to be present in a black person than in a white person.

In our previous discussion of diagnostic tests, we showed that the lower the prevalence rate in a population (i.e., the rarer the disease) the lower the predictive value of a positive test. For a rare disease, then, a positive test is much less likely to indicate disease. Clinicians automatically and perhaps subconsciously employ this concept. They know that a young woman with t wave changes on an electrocardiogram is unlikely to have coronary artery disease. They know that a young man with persistent abdominal pain is unlikely to have pancreatic cancer. They know that a white person with evidence of joint pain and anemia is still unlikely to have sickle-cell anemia. The clinician's appreciation of the rates of the disease may be based entirely on clinical experience; however, it is helpful to be able to draw from research articles to gain a more objective and scientific assessment of the rates of disease. This section will aim at assisting the reader to acquire the tools to understand how the rates of disease are scientifically measured and interpreted. Such an understanding helps one to choose the proper diagnostic methods more thoughtfully and to gain insight from the choices made.

In addition to facilitating individual diagnosis, an appreciation of the rates of illness helps in the assessment of changes that occur over time or as a result of medical intervention. Rates of illness are an important tool for conducting the types of studies that were discussed in Part 1. The ability to identify real changes and true cause and effect relationships is dependent on an understanding of the principles of comparing rates.

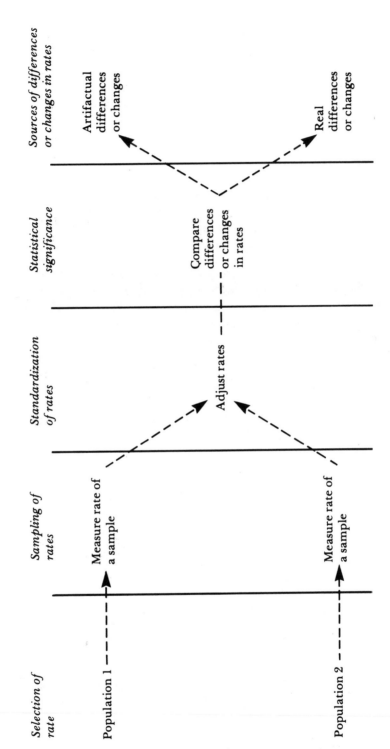

FIGURE 18-1. Uniform framework for Rating a Rate.

154

A uniform framework made up of the following components should assist the reader in understanding how rates are developed and used.

SELECTION OF RATES   Defining different types of rates

SAMPLING OF RATES   Defining the methods for obtaining estimates of rates by studying only a portion of the population

STANDARDIZATION OF RATES   Comparing rates after taking into account differences in the populations

STATISTICAL SIGNIFICANCE OF RATES   Determining the probability of obtaining the observed differences in rates if there is no true difference in rates in the larger populations from which the sample rates are drawn

SOURCES OF DIFFERENCES OR CHANGES IN RATES   Distinguishing real from artifactual differences or changes in rates. Artifactual changes or differences are those that are attributable to change in the way a disease is defined or measured.

Figure 18-1 summarizes the uniform framework for rating a rate.

It may not be obvious why it is necessary to study the rates of disease. Why not just compare how many times events occur? Let us look at the following example, which illustrates the problems with comparing only the number of events that occur.

A hospital review panel was evaluating the performance of physicians at your hospital. They found that you had five deaths among the 1,000 patients you treated at the hospital last year. The Chief of Staff had only one death among the 200 patients he treated. The panel decided that since you had five times the number of deaths as the Chief of Staff you must have been practicing bad medicine.

You don't have to be prepared to defend yourself by saying, "It might look bad, but I'm really OK!" Instead of looking at the total number of deaths, it is fairer to look at the number of deaths that occurred in relation to the number of deaths that could have occurred. You merely need to point out that your death rate and the Chief of Staff's were identical: 5 per 1,000 equals 1 per 200. Rates of events have come to your defense. They're worth knowing about!

An important use of rates in clinical medicine is their role in evaluating the risk or probability of developing a disease. In assessing risk, one must know how many times the disease could have occurred. One must know how many individuals were "at risk" of developing the disease as well as how many actually developed the disease. In other words:

$$\text{Risk of development of a disease} = \frac{\text{Number of times the disease occurs over a period of time}}{\text{Number of individuals in the at risk population over the same period of time}}$$

Unfortunately, it is often difficult to estimate how many individuals could have developed the disease over a period of time because a population is constantly changing as individuals move in, move out, or die. To circumvent this problem, the concept of rate is frequently substituted for the concept of risk. A rate differs from a risk in that the denominator of a rate includes only those individuals who are at risk of developing the disease at one point in time, ideally, at the midpoint of the time period of interest. Thus a definition of the rate of development of a disease would be constructed this way:

$$\text{Rate of development of a disease} = \frac{\text{Number of times the disease occurs over a period of time}}{\text{Number of individuals in the at risk population at mid-point of the time period of interest}}$$

If, for instance, one wanted to study the probability of developing a duodenal ulcer in New York City in 1980, the risk would be calculated as follows:

$$\text{Risk of developing duodenal ulcer in New York City in 1980} = \frac{\text{Number of New York City residents who developed duodenal ulcer in 1980}}{\text{Number of New York City residents at risk of developing duodenal ulcer during 1980}}$$

Since individuals are constantly moving in or out of New York City, it is difficult to know the true number of persons who lived in the city during 1980. Since a census is available for New York City on April 1, 1980, however, one could use this point of time to calculate a rate instead of a risk. The rate of duodenal ulcers in New York City in 1980 then would be calculated as follows:

$$\text{Rate of developing duodenal ulcer in New York City in 1980} = \frac{\text{Number of New York City residents who developed duodenal ulcer in 1980}}{\substack{\text{Number of New York City residents at risk}\\ \text{of developing duodenal ulcer on April 1, 1980}\\ \text{(about equal to the number of New York City}\\ \text{residents on April 1, 1980)}}}$$

Fortunately, the rate of events is a good approximation of the risk of developing a disease unless the disease is extremely frequent *and* is rapidly fatal, which eliminates individuals from the population. Only if both these conditions are met would the population at risk in New York City on April 1, 1980 be much different from the population at risk during 1980. However, for practical purposes, one may equate the rate of development of a disease with the risk of development of the disease.

The type of rate we have been talking about here is an *incidence* rate, which is an approximation of the risk of developing a disease. The incidence rate measures the new cases of a particular disease that develop over a defined period of time. Once a disease does occur, it may be present for a long period of time. Thus, a second rate frequently is used, which estimates the risk of *having* a disease at a point in time. Known as the *prevalence* rate, it measures how frequent or prevalent the disease is at any one point in time. The prevalence rate of disease is very important in diagnosis since it estimates the probability of disease. It provides an estimate of the likelihood of the presence of disease before evaluating an individual's history, physical examination, or laboratory tests. Thus,

$$\text{Prevalence rate} = \frac{\text{Number of individuals who have the disease at a point in time}}{\text{Number of individuals who are in the population at the same point in time}}$$

The previous example of the prevalence rate of duodenal ulcers on April 1, 1980 in New York City then would be constructed as follows:

$$\text{Prevalence rate} = \frac{\text{Number of New York City residents with duodenal ulcer on April 1, 1980}}{\text{Number of New York City residents on April 1, 1980}}$$

The prevalence rate has a defined relationship to the incidence rate, thus,

Prevalence rate = incidence rate × duration of the disease

In other words, the longer the average duration of the disease, the more individuals will have the disease at any particular time, therefore the higher the prevalence rate. Chronic diseases with long duration, such as diabetes, may have a lower incidence of development of new cases but a higher prevalence of the disease at any point in time. Acute, short-duration diseases like strep throat may have a high incidence of occurrence of new cases but a low prevalence of the disease at any point in time. Thus it is important to appreciate that incidence rates and prevalence rates measure different phenomena. Incidence rates measure the probability of *developing* a new case of the disease. Prevalence rates measure the probability of *having* the disease at a particular time. Failure to appreciate this difference may lead to the type of error illustrated in the following example.

A study of gonorrhea in males was conducted by taking cultures from 10,000 randomly selected males. Of the 100 males diagnosed as having gonorrhea, the study found that 15 were asymptomatic for a rate of asymptomatic infection of 15%. A related study was performed by following up the male partners of women newly diagnosed as having gonorrhea. 100 males with gonorrhea were identified, but only two were asymptomatic for an asymptomatic rate of only 2%. In comparing these studies a reviewer concluded that one of them must be in error since the conclusions were so widely divergent.

This seeming inconsistency is not inconsistent at all if one distinguishes incidence rates from prevalence rates. The first study, which cultured 10,000 males at a particular point in time, produced a prevalence rate. The second study, which followed up new cases of gonorrhea, was an incidence study. The fact that the prevalence rate of asymptomatic gonorrhea was much higher than the incidence rate suggests that asymptomatic cases have a long duration. This may be explained by the fact that symptomatic cases are treated and cured while asymptomatic cases remain in the population for long periods of time, producing higher prevalence rates.

Under some circumstances, it is possible to determine every case of a disease in a population. Death rates usually can be obtained on entire populations because death certificates are mandatory legal documents. It is often possible therefore to obtain the complete rates of death from a disease for an entire population. For most diseases, however, it is not feasible to count every case of the disease in an entire population, in which instance the techniques of sampling are very helpful. Sampling ideally means that an investigator randomly selects only a portion of the population, studies this sample, and then tries to extrapolate the results to the entire population that was intended for study.

The Standard Error

Even when properly performed, the process of sampling is not perfect. To appreciate the process of sampling and the inherent error introduced by sampling, one must understand the basic principle that underlies sampling techniques. This principle states that if many random samples of a rate are obtained, the sample rates on the average will be the same as the rate of the original population. In other words, each sample may differ from the original population either by having a higher rate or a lower rate. However, for every sample that is one unit above the rate of the original population, there will be one sample that is the same distance below that rate. Therefore, on the average, the sample rates will be the same as the rate for the original population. For example, if the original population has a rate of 1 per 100,

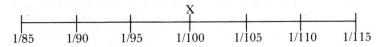

and if the samples were taken from this original population, the rates might look like this:

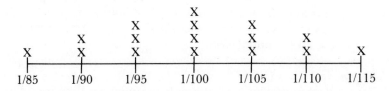

Notice that while some of the sample rates are equal to the rate of the original population, many of them are either higher or lower. Because samples are accurate only on the average, a single sample is said to possess an inherent sampling error. Statistical methods are available to measure the likely size of the error. The statistical measure—known as the standard error—attempts to estimate from the sample the size of this error due to sampling.

This standard error has the important property that 95% of the time the true value of the population will fall within a range of two standard errors above and two standard errors below the sample's value. Therefore, if a sample value is 5% ± 1%, 95% of the time one can say with assurance that the true value for the population lies between 3% and 7%. This range is known as the 95% confidence limit and provides the best estimate that can be obtained from the sample for the true value in the larger population. Failure to take into account this range of values can produce the following misinterpretation.

A national organization attempted to estimate the rate of strep carriers by culturing a random sample of 0.1% of all the school children in the nation. To verify their results, the same organization used a second random sample of 0.1% of the nation's schools and simultaneously conducted a second survey using an indentical protocol. The first survey revealed a rate of 15 per 1,000 positive strep cultures while the second survey revealed a rate of 10 per 1,000. The authors concluded that the inconsistent results were impossible since they had used the same methodology.

The authors failed to state or to take into account the fact that samples have an inherent error. To deal with the error, the authors should have calculated the standard errors of these estimates. It is possible that the 95% confidence limits would have been large enough to make the results of these studies completely compatible. This example merely points out that two identically conducted samples may produce different results on the basis of chance alone. Remember that large numbers of samples, on the average, produce values identical with the true value for the population, but that any two samples may vary widely from one another and from the true value in the larger population.

Sample Size
There is a second important principle in understanding sampling. This principle says that the more individuals who are included in

a sample, the more likely the sample's rate will closely approximate the rate in the larger population. Notice that it is not the number of samples obtained, but the size of the particular sample that determines how close the sample rate is likely to be to the rate of the larger population.

Let us look more closely at this principle. The size of the standard error measures how well the sample estimates the true value in the larger population. The major factor affecting the size of the standard error is the size of the sample. The relationship between sample size and accuracy is not one to one; it is a square root function. With small sample sizes, increasing the size of the sample may greatly increase the accuracy of the sample. As the sample gets larger, however, the returns diminish and small or moderate increases in sample size may add little to the accuracy of the estimate. Investigators therefore attempt to balance the need for accuracy against the financial costs of increasing the sample size. The consequence of using small sample sizes is that the samples may vary widely from one sample to another and from the true value in the larger population. The following example illustrates the need to take into account the effects of sample size on the results of sampling.

An investigator who sampled 0.1% of the nation's hospitals concluded that the rate of diagnosis of pancreatic cancer was 50 per 100,000 ± 20 per year. A second investigator who sampled 1% of the nation's hospitals concluded that the true value for the nation was 80 per 100,000 ± 5 per year. The second investigator concluded that the first study was performed fraudulently since it had a much wider range of possible values.

The first study used a sample size only one-tenth as great as the second study; it is not surprising therefore that the standard error of the first study was much larger, that is, 20 versus 5. In the first study the range of possible values was $50 \pm 2\ (20) = 10$ to 90 per 100,000. Notice that the range of values includes 80, the value found in the second study. The wider range of possible values for the larger population in the first study is not necessarily a result of errors in the study; it is a natural consequence of the smaller sample size used.

Random Sampling
Having outlined two important principles of sampling, there is one further point to consider. These two principles rest on the as-

sumption that the sampling has been randomly obtained, meaning that all individuals in the population have an equal chance of being chosen for inclusion in the sample. Unless random sampling is performed, one cannot accurately estimate how close the sample results are to those of the larger population. The need for random sampling is illustrated in the following example.

An investigator from one county hospital estimated that the community rate of myocardial infarction was 150 per 100,000 per year. An investigator at a private hospital in the same community estimated that the rate was 155 per 100,000 per year. Since their results were similar the investigators concluded that the rate of myocardial infarctions in their community must be between 150 and 155 per 100,000 per year.

Neither of these studies attempted to obtain a random sample of the larger community population. It is possible that myocardial infarction patients either selectively chose these two hospitals or were selectively sent to them. If all the area hospitals were included in the sample, the rate of myocardial infarction might have been quite different. The rates in this example were calculated from conveniently available data known as "chunk sampling." It is the simplest sampling to perform since the investigators merely calculate the rates for an easily available population. The nonrepresentativeness of a chunk sample, however, means that it cannot be easily or reliably extrapolated to the larger population.

Despite the statistical desirability of random sampling, many investigators have found that, if they rely exclusively on random sampling, they will fail to include enough individuals who possess the characteristics of interest for their study. For instance, if investigators are studying the rates of hypertension in the United States, they may also be interested in the rates of hypertension for blacks or orientals. If they merely took a random sample of the population, it may not include very many blacks or orientals. Therefore, investigators would separately sample from blacks, from orientals, and from the rest of the population. This separate sampling from the different subsets or strata of the population is known as stratified sampling. It is permissible to do separate or stratified sampling as long as the sampling within each group is random. There are separate statistical methods for use with stratified samples. They also result in standard errors that estimate the possible range of true values for the rates in the larger populations.

Let us review the principles and requirements for sampling.

1. On the average, samples drawn from a population will have the same rate as the original population. There is however an inherent error introduced by sampling. This error can be estimated by calculating the standard error of the sample.

2. The size of the standard error is affected by the size of the sample obtained. Increasing the sample size decreases the size of the standard error, but diminishing returns set in as one increases the size of the sample.

3. The principles of sampling rest on the assumption that samples are randomly obtained. It is permissible to assure adequate numbers in each category of interest by stratified sampling. However, sampling must be random within each category or stratum. If random sampling is not performed there is no way of accurately relating the rate obtained to the true rate of the larger population.

In the previous chapter we outlined the requirements for accurately obtaining rates using random sampling. Here, we will attempt to compare the rates once they are obtained. We will assume that the rates have been properly obtained and illustrate the precautions that must be observed in comparing rates, even those that are measured using proper random sampling techniques.

We will be comparing rates from two different populations. These populations may be two hospitals, two cities, two countries, two factories, or the same population compared at different points in time. We will be comparing rates to determine the size of the difference in rates or the extent of change in the rates. This comparison is important for rates derived from sampling as well as for rates determined by using the entire population.

When using rates to compare risks of disease, it is important to consider whether the populations differ by a factor that is already known to affect the risk of the disease. This consideration is parallel with the adjustment for confounding variables discussed previously.

In performing a study, the investigator may know already that factors such as age, sex or race affect the rate of developing a particular disease. At the same time, the investigator may want to determine if the rates would differ if these factors were taken into account; thus the investigator would then adjust for, or "standardize" the rates for these factors. The importance of standardization can be seen if the rates of lung cancer in a college community are compared to a retirement community. If one knows already that age affects the rate of lung cancer, little is gained by discovering that the retirement community has a higher rate of lung cancer. Likewise, if one factory has a younger work force than a second factory, it is unfair to compare the lung cancer rates directly, especially if the attempt is made to draw conclusions about the safety of working conditions.

To circumvent this problem, rates of disease can be adjusted to take into account the factors that are already known to greatly affect the risk of illness. This process of adjustment of rates is known as *standardization*. Age is the most common factor that requires standardization, but any factor known to have a large effect can be *adjusted for*. For instance, using the techniques of standardization in comparing the rates of hypertension in two populations, one might adjust for race since blacks are known to have a higher rate of hypertension.

The principle used in standardizing rates is the same as that used to adjust for the differences in study populations discussed in Chapter 5. Investigators aim to compare rates, for instance, for individuals who are similar in age or any other factor that is being adjusted. Before illustrating the method used for adjustment, let us see just how misleading results can be if standardization is not performed.

The incidence of pancreatic cancer in the United States was compared to the incidence of the same cancer in Mexico. The rate in the U.S. was found to be three times the rate in Mexico per 100,000 population. The authors concluded that Americans are at three times greater risk of pancreatic cancer than Mexicans, assuming that the accuracy of diagnosis and estimate of population were equal in the two countries.

The interpretation of this study is superficially correct; the risk of pancreatic cancer is higher in the U.S. if the data here are reliable. However the average age of the Mexican population is much younger than in the United States. It may be that the younger age of the Mexican population accounts for the difference in rates of pancreatic cancer since increased age is known to be associated with increased pancreatic cancer. If the age distribution does not explain these differences, then the investigators may have detected an important unexpected difference that requires further explanation. The authors should standardize their data for age and see if the differences persist.

The usual method for standardization of rates, known as the direct method, works as follows. Suppose investigators wish to compare the rates of bladder cancer in two large industries. The bladder cancer data for the two industries are shown in Table 21-1. Notice that the overall rates for both populations are 200 per 100,000 workers. Also, notice that the rates for each age group are as high or higher in factory A than in factory B. Despite the lower rates for each age group at factory B, it may at first seem surprising that the overall rates are the same. However, looking at the number of individuals in each age group, it becomes apparent that factory A has a much younger work force than factory B. Factory B has 60,000 workers from age 50 to 70 while factory A has only 30,000 workers in these age groups. Since bladder cancer is known to

TABLE 21-1. COMPARISON OF RATES OF BLADDER CANCER

FACTORY A

Age	Number of individuals	Number of cases of bladder cancer	Rate of bladder cancer in each age group*
20–30	20,000	0	0 per 100,000
30–40	20,000	10	50 per 100,000
40–50	30,000	20	67 per 100,000
50–60	20,000	80	400 per 100,000
60–70	10,000	90	900 per 100,000
Total	100,000	200	200 per 100,000

FACTORY B

Age	Number of individuals	Number of cases of bladder cancer	Rate of bladder cancer in each age group*
20–30	10,000	0	0 per 100,000
30–40	10,000	4	40 per 100,000
40–50	20,000	6	30 per 100,000
50–60	50,000	140	280 per 100,000
60–70	10,000	50	500 per 100,000
Total	100,000	200	200 per 100,000

*The rate is obtained from the number of cases and the number of individuals in the age group. The rates cannot be added down the column.

increase with age, the younger age of factory A's work force reduced the overall rates in factory A. Thus, it is unfair to factory B to look only at the overall rates since factory B's overall rate is increased by its older population. This is especially true if we are asking questions about the safety of the factory environment itself.

To avoid this problem, the authors must standardize the rates to adjust for the differences in age and thereby compare the rates more fairly. To accomplish standardization, each population is subdivided to indicate the number of individuals, the number of cases

TABLE 21-2. METHOD OF AGE STANDARDIZATION

Age group	Rate of bladder cancer in factory A	Number of individuals in factory B	Number of cases that would occur in factory A if it had the same age distribution as factory B*	Number of cases of bladder cancer that actually occurred in factory B
20–30	0/100,000	10,000	0	0
30–40	50/100,000	10,000	5	4
40–50	67/100,000	20,000	13	6
50–60	400/100,000	50,000	200	140
60–70	900/100,000	10,000	90	50
Totals		100,000	308	200

*This column is calculated by multiplying the previous two columns.

of the disease, and the rate in each age group. This has been done already and is shown in Table 21-1.

The authors then must attempt to determine how many cases of bladder cancer would have occurred in factory A if the age distribution were the same as in factory B. The steps in this process are as follows.

1. Starting with the 20 to 30 age group, the authors take the rate of cancer for that group in factory A and multiply this by the number of individuals in the corresponding age group in factory B. This produces the number of cases that would have occurred in factory A if it had the same number of individuals in that age group as factory B.

2. The authors then perform this calculation for each age group and add up the total number of cases from the different age groups. This produces a total number of cases which would have occurred if factory A had the same overall age distribution as factory B.

3. The authors now have standardized the rates for age and can

compare directly the number of cases that occurred in factory B with the number of cases that would have occurred in factory A if factory A had the same age distribution as factory B.

Let us apply these procedures to the bladder cancer data as shown in Table 21-2.

Three hundred and eight cases of bladder cancer would have occurred in factory A while only 200 actually did occur in factory B. These figures are a better measure for comparing the risk to the workers of developing bladder cancer in each factory. The numbers accentuate the fact that despite the equality of the overall rates, factory A has a rate as high or higher in each age group. Therefore, in order to make fair comparisons between populations where age is known to affect the risk of disease, it is necessary to age-standardize the populations. If additional factors also are known greatly to affect the rates, the same process can be applied to standardize or adjust for these factors.

Statistical Significance
of Rates

If the entire population is used to derive the rates, then one knows that the observed differences or changes are not the result of sampling errors. However, if sampling was employed to derive the rates, then one is interested in knowing whether the differences or changes are statistically significant. By performing a statistical significance test, one is asking what the probability is of obtaining the observed or greater differences in the sample rates if there are no true differences in the larger populations.

In addition to formulating a hypothesis and collecting the data the following steps occur.

1. The investigator assumes the null hypothesis that no difference between the rates exists in the larger populations.

2. The investigator determines the probability or significance level that will be considered so small that the investigator will reject the null hypothesis and accept by elimination the conclusion that a true difference in rates exists in the larger populations. *Small* is usually defined as 5% or less.

3. Using statistical methods the investigator calculates the probability that the observed difference in the rates could have occurred by chance if no true difference exists in the larger populations.

4. If the probability that the observed differences in the rates could have occurred by chance is equal to or less than 5%, the authors can reject the null hypothesis and accept by elimination the conclusion that true differences in rates exist in the larger populations.

The process of comparing the two rates is simplified when the rates are reported with standard errors. The interval, two standard errors above or below a sample's rate, tells one with 95% confidence where the true rate for the larger population lies. These confidence limits have another important property with randomly sampled rates. The confidence limits provide a convenient method for determining whether the difference in the two rates is likely to be statistically significant. If one sample's rate lies outside the 95% confidence limit of the other sample, then a statistically significant difference exists.

For instance, imagine that a study sampled the rates for congenital heart defects in male versus female infants. The rate in males was 50 per 100,000 ± 10 while the rate among females was 80 per 100,000 ± 12. This means that the sample's rate for males was found to be 50 per 100,000 and one standard error was 10 per 100,000. Likewise, the observed rate for females was 80 per 100,000 and one standard error equals 12 per 100,000. The reader may want to rapidly compare these rates to know whether the differences are statistically significant. This comparison is shown in Figure 22-1.

Notice that the confidence limits overlap but neither confidence limit reaches the value obtained in the other sample. This simple graphic representation can rapidly tell you if the differences in the two rates are statistically significant. The importance of considering the statistical significance of differences and reporting the standard errors is illustrated in the following example.

A well conducted study of the rate of malignant melanoma was performed by random sampling of all the hospitals in the nation. The authors discovered that the rates of malignant melanoma were as follows:

1976: 15 per 100,000 ± 3
1977: 10 per 100,000 ± 3
1978: 15 per 100,000 ± 3

The authors concluded that a condition must have existed in 1977 that reduced the rate of disease. This example illustrates the importance of knowing the confidence limits around each rate. The confidence limits are wide enough around the 1977 rate to also include the 1976 and 1978 rates. Thus the differences may only have reflected chance sampling errors and may not represent true differences.

The possibility of Type I and Type II errors always exists with statistical significance testing. Remember that it is possible to decrease the size of the standard errors and consequently reduce the range of the confidence limits by increasing the size of the samples. Even when it has not been possible to show that a true difference exists, a difference may well exist and could be demonstrated if larger numbers were used. Studies with a very large number of individuals allow one to detect very small, even inconsequential differences in rates in the larger population.

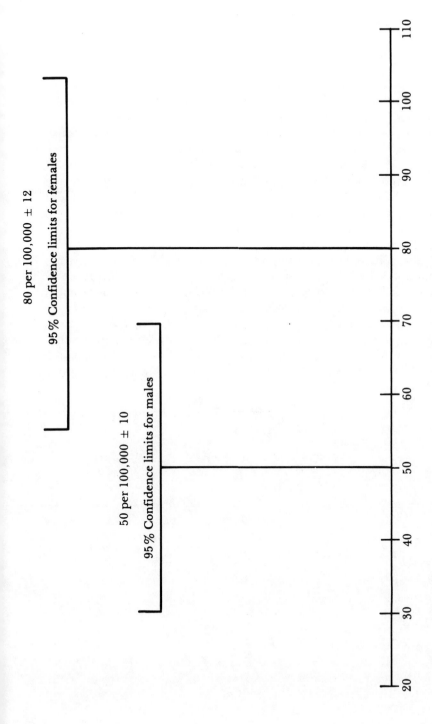

FIGURE 22-1. The 95% confidence limits surrounding the congenital heart defect rates for males and females.

The previous discussion of statistical significance is applicable only when rates are determined by random sampling. Samples introduce inherent but measurable errors. If, on the other hand, entire populations are compared, then no sampling errors exist. It is then possible to directly compare the rates to see if a difference exists. For instance, in the bladder cancer example in Chapter 21, the entire population of each factory was used to calculate the rates. It was possible therefore to directly compare the rates without the need for statistical significance tests. Only standardization needed to be performed to fairly compare rates.

Thus, it is possible to assess whether a difference in rates is present by either including the entire population and comparing the rates directly or by sampling the rates and using the proof by elimination method of statistical significance testing. It is essential to remember that statistically significant differences are not necessarily clinically important differences. When a difference is large enough to be of potential importance, one should try to understand the source of this difference. Does it represent a real change or is it the result of changes in the way a disease is defined or measured? This is the topic of the next chapter.

Sources of Differences in Rates

In this chapter, let us assume that it has been established that two populations have differences in rates. These differences may have been shown by measurements of rates using the entire population or by sampling rates and determining whether a statistically significant difference exists. Differences between rates may represent differences between two populations or differences over time in the same population.

Artifactual Differences or Changes

The differences in rates may be the result of real changes or they may reflect changes or differences in the means by which the disease under consideration is defined or measured. Artifactual differences imply that, despite the fact that a difference exists, the difference is not a reflection of changes in the disease but merely in the way the disease is defined or measured.

Artifactual changes are of three types:

1. Changes in the *ability* to recognize the disease. These represent changes in the measurement of the disease.
2. Changes in the *efforts* to recognize disease. These may represent efforts to recognize the disease at an earlier stage, changes in reporting requirements or new incentives to search for the disease.
3. Changes in the *definition* of the disease. These represent changes in the terminology used to define the disease.

The following example illustrates the first type of artifactual change, the effect of a change in the ability to recognize a disease.

Because of a recent increase in interest, a study of the prevalence of mitral valve prolapse was performed. A complete survey of the charts at a major university cardiac clinic found that in 1967 only 1 per 1,000 patients had a diagnosis of mitral valve prolapse, while in 1981, 80 per 1,000 had mitral valve prolapse included in their diagnosis. The authors concluded that the condition was increasing at an astounding rate.

Between 1967 and 1981 the use of echocardiography greatly increased the ability to document mitral valve prolapse. In addition, the growing recognition of the frequency of this condition led to

177

a much better understanding of how to recognize it by physical examination. It is not surprising then that a much larger proportion of cardiac clinic patients were known to have mitral valve prolapse in 1981 compared to 1967. It is possible that if an equal understanding and equal technology were available in 1967, the rates would have been nearly identical. This example demonstrates that artifactual changes may explain large differences in the rates of disease even when a complete review of all cases is used to accurately calculate the rate of disease.

Changes in the efforts to recognize disease may occur when physicians attempt to diagnose disease at an earlier stage. If a screening program is introduced to diagnose a disease at a stage when no symptoms exist, then individuals are likely to be diagnosed sooner. The efforts at earlier diagnosis produce a "lead-time" in diagnosis compared to the previous method. If the available treatment is more successful when applied earlier, then this may result in an improved outlook or prognosis. If, however, there is no adequate treatment or early treatment makes no difference, then one may be merely increasing the interval between diagnosis and death. It may produce an artifactual difference if the rate of death is measured in the immediate time period after diagnosis. An example of the effect of increased lead-time is illustrated in the following example.

Prior to the introduction of an X-ray screening program for lung cancer, the six-month mortality rate was 80 deaths per 100 cases of lung cancer diagnosed. After the introduction of the screening program, the six-month mortality rate was 20 per 100 diagnosed cases. The authors concluded that the screening program had drastically lowered the early death rate from lung cancer and thus had proved its value.

The screening program probably diagnosed cases of lung cancer at an asymptomatic stage versus the previous diagnosis that occurred after symptoms were present. However, there is evidence that suggests the long-term prognosis of lung cancer is not altered by X-ray screening. X-ray screening probably merely alters the lead-time between diagnosis and death. Thus the observed changes are probably artifactual due to the earlier recognition of the disease.

The following example illustrates how the meaning of terminology may change over time and thus produce an artifactual change in the rate of events.

A study of candidates for hemodialysis showed that in 1965, 50% of the patients in a major metropolitan area with chronic renal failure were considered "acceptable candidates for hemodialysis." In 1980 the percentage of patients with chronic renal failure in the same community who were considered "acceptable candidates" had risen to 95%. The authors concluded that the nature of the disease process in the community had changed.

Between 1965 and 1980 there was an enormous expansion in the financial support for renal hemodialysis and in the ability to perform the procedure. As facilities, finances, and interest in doing dialysis expanded, it is possible that the definition of an "acceptable candidate" changed. It is more likely that changes in the definition of "acceptable candidate" rather than changes in the nature of the disease process led to the change in rates. This is an example of how changes in definition may produce an artifactual change in rates.

Real Changes

Artifactual changes in rates imply that the true incidence or prevalence of rates has not been altered even though an apparent change in rates has occurred. Real changes, however, imply that the incidence or prevalence rates have actually changed. One first must ask whether any of the sources of artifactual differences are operating. If they are not operating or are not large enough to explain the differences, one can assume that real differences or changes exist. There are a series of sources for these real changes—each of which carries a different meaning and therefore different implications. The study of real changes or differences in rates is an attempt to understand why true changes in rates have occurred over time or why two populations have different rates. The study of real changes may provide insight into the causes or prevention of a disease.

The first type of real change that can occur is a change in the prognosis or life expectancy once the disease is diagnosed. An improvement in prognosis, however, cannot be expected to affect the rate of development of a new disease as measured by the incidence rate. The prevalence rate equals the incidence rate times the average duration of disease. Thus, improved survival without cure often keeps more individuals with the disease alive and may even increase the prevalence rate as illustrated in the following example.

In a study of the rates of duodenal ulcer disease, the authors properly obtained the death rate from duodenal ulcers for the United States in 1940 and 1975. In 1940, the rate of death from duodenal ulcer was 5 per 1,000,000 while in 1975 it was 1 per 1,000,000. They also found that the incidence rate had not changed and the prevalence rates had increased slightly. They concluded that these findings were inconsistent and did not provide any information on what had happened.

The change observed may well have reflected real changes in the mortality or death rates due to duodenal ulcer. The fact that the incidence rates had not changed suggests that individuals continued to develop duodenal ulcer, but once it developed, the prognosis or outlook was better in 1975 than in 1940. A lowering of the proportion who die from a disease may increase the prevalence rate by extending the duration of disease. The improved prognosis has not affected the incidence of new disease and has slightly increased the prevalence rate. These changes are consistent.

A second type of real change may result from the unusual circumstances that may have existed at the start of a study of rates. It is not unusual for a study to be initiated because of the suspicion that the rates of events are increasing. Investigators may believe that the frequency of cancer, heart disease, influenza, or venereal disease is on the rise. Changes in rates over a short period of time may have at least three possible explanations: (1) These changes may herald future changes in the same direction; (2) they may reflect predictable cycles or epidemics; (3) they may be the result of unpredictable chance fluctuations representing an unusual frequency of events. Before concluding that observed changes in rates are likely to continue, one must consider the possibility either of cyclical or chance fluctuations. If there is a natural cycle in the frequency of the disease, the rate from year to year may look like Figure 23-1.

If investigators should note the increase that occurred between 1973 and 1974, they may attempt to measure the changes between 1974 and 1976 and would again find an increase. It is important,

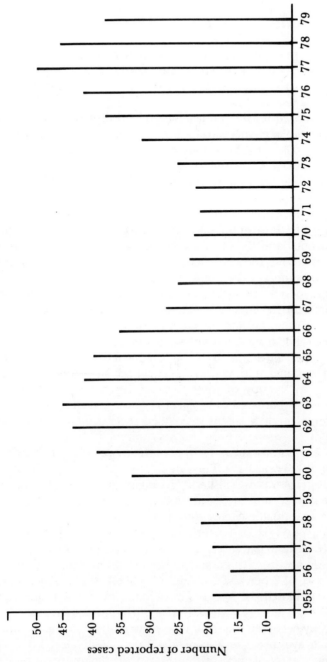

FIGURE 23-1. Predictable cycles or epidemics in the yearly incidence of a disease.

181

however, that investigators realize that this real change between 1974 and 1976 may be part of the natural cycle of disease. It does not necessarily imply that a further increase can be expected in 1977, 1978 or 1979.

As opposed to this predictable cycle of disease, there may be an unpredictable, chance variation in the rate of disease from year to year (Fig. 23-2) In this situation if investigators pick a year where the rate was higher and compare it to the next year where by chance alone the rate was lower, they may believe they are documenting important changes when, in fact, they are merely discovering the principle of *regression to the mean*. Regression to the mean or return to the average states that unusual values are by definition rare events, and the odds are against a repetition of a rare event twice in a row. In fact, by chance alone, the next measurement is likely to be nearer the average value.

Regression to the mean may occur because of the natural chance fluctuation of events or it may occur because of forces that react to the unusual rate and force it into line or back toward the average or mean. For instance, if one were studying how much an individual eats per meal, it is likely that the meal following an indulgence would be smaller than usual. Let us see how this principle may operate in a study of rates that produced real differences, but differences that need to be carefully interpreted.

After a tragic accident that killed several men in a factory, an accident prevention program was initiated. Investigators found that the accident rate at the time of the tragedy was unusually high, 10 per 1,000 workdays. The rate fell to 2 per 1,000 workdays when the program was established. The investigators concluded that the accident prevention program was an enormous success.

The investigators have shown that a real change took place. They have not, however, shown that it was the accident prevention program that caused the change. It is possible that the 10 per 1,000 rate was unusually high and by chance alone returned to a more usual rate of 2 per 1,000. Even more likely, the fatal accident may have frightened the workers into taking more safety precautions. The authors started with an unusually high accident rate and then a tragedy occurred that could have forced the rate back toward the mean or average. The authors documented a true change but one that may be explained by regression to the mean rather than a long-lasting change.

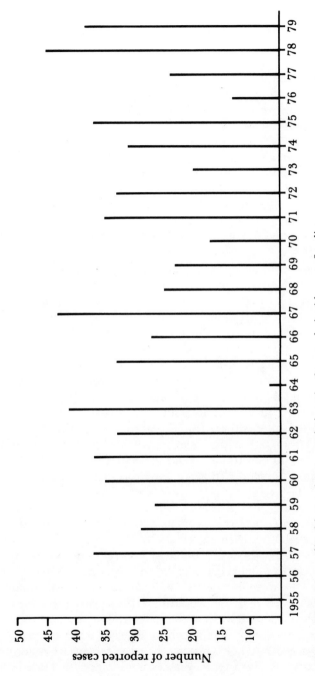

FIGURE 23-2. Unpredictable or chance variations in the yearly incidence of a disease.

It is important to recognize the phenomenon of regression to the mean because it may be operating whenever short-term changes in rates are observed. It is premature to conclude that the accident prevention program would help other groups or even this group if it were done at another time. Thus, the principle of regression to the mean may be the source of real changes in rates, but this source of real changes may have limited importance and may imply that observed changes are not guaranteed to continue.

A third source of real differences is known as the *cohort effect*. A cohort is a group of individuals who share a common experience or exposure. If one or several cohorts in a population have undergone an exposure or experience that makes them particularly susceptible to disease, then the possibility of a cohort effect exists. The rates for the age group, which includes the susceptible cohort, thus may be temporarily increased. This temporary increase is known as the cohort effect. When a cohort effect is present, one can expect the rates for this particular age group to fall again as time passes and the susceptible cohort passes beyond this particular age group. The importance of appreciating the cohort effect is illustrated in the following example.

An investigator was studying the rates of thyroid cancer. Concern existed that past pediatric head and neck radiation frequently used before 1950 was a contributor to thyroid cancers. Using proper methods, the authors found that the rate of thyroid cancer among the 20- to 30-year age group in 1950 was 50 per 100,000, in 1960 it was 100 per 100,000, and in 1970 it was 150 per 100,000. The authors concluded that by 1980 the rates would pass the 200 per 100,000 mark.

The authors have established that real changes were occurring in the rates of thyroid cancer in the 20- to 30-year age group. The source of these changes may be a cohort effect. The cohort of individuals who were radiated before 1950 carried an increased risk of thyroid cancer that did not necessarily affect those individuals who were born after 1950. By 1980, all individuals in the 20- to 30-year age group would have been born after 1950. Thus, one might have seen a fall in the 1980 thyroid cancer rate in 20- to 30-year-olds rather than a continued rise. The concept of a cohort effect not only helps predict the expected future rates, it also helps to support the theory that past radiation increased the risk of thyroid cancer. If a fall in the rate occurred as predicted for 1980, this would further support the theory.

The cohort effect is another source which helps to explain the cause of real changes in rates. The cohort effect, by isolating the changes to one segment of the population, helps to predict future rates better than mere extrapolation from the observed changes.

In summary, to analyze differences or changes in rates, it is necessary to determine whether a difference in rates is artifactual or real. If artifactual changes have been excluded, it is worthwhile to try to understand the source of real differences.

Summary: Rating a Rate

Let us review the steps required for development, comparison, and interpretation of rates of disease. The following summary, is organized according to our uniform framework for rating a rate.

Selection of Rates

Incidence rates are important clinical measures since they approximate the risk of *developing* disease over a period of time. Prevalence rates help in diagnosis by approximating the risk of *having* a disease at a particular point in time. Readers must distinguish between these two types of rates.

Sampling of Rates

Rates may be derived by using the entire, larger population. Alternatively, rates can be calculated using only samples of the larger population. The sample rates, on the average, are the same as the larger population, but any one sample possesses an inherent error statistically expressed by the standard error. The larger the size of the sample, the smaller the standard error. However, returns diminish for large samples and the investigators must weigh accuracy against cost. The ability to estimate the rate of a large population from a sample requires random sampling from the larger population. It is possible to stratify the sample to assure large enough numbers in each category, but sampling must be random within each category.

Standardization of Rates

Whether obtained by inclusion of the entire population or by sampling, one is interested in comparing rates to assess the differences between populations or changes over time. When comparing rates, a fair comparison often requires that the rates be adjusted for factors known to affect the rate of disease, which are different in the two populations. Demographic factors such as age, sex, and race are frequently adjusted for or standardized in order to look for other factors which produce the differences or changes in rates.

Statistical Significance

If the entire population was used to derive the rates, then one knows that the observed differences or changes actually occurred. However, if sampling was employed, one wants to know whether the differences are statistically significant. A statistically significant change or difference implies there is a low probability of obtaining the observed data if there are no true differences between the larger populations. Statistical significance alone says little about the size or importance of the differences found.

Sources of Changes or Differences

The meaning of the differences is assessed by examining the differences to determine whether they are artifactual or real. Changes in ability to recognize the disease, efforts to recognize the disease, or definition of the disease may produce artifactual changes or differences that are of little clinical importance.

If no artifactual changes have occurred or they could not explain the differences, then a real difference or change is assumed to be present. Real changes may result from changes in the prognosis of a disease once developed. These changes will not alter the incidence rate directly. It is important to recognize a second type of real fluctuation or change in rates known as regression to the mean. This effect often occurs when the original rate used for comparison is unusual. This unusual rate may set forces in motion that help bring the future rates back toward or even below the average. Alternatively, chance alone may produce a subsequent rate, which is much closer to the mean or the average.

A third type of real change in rates is known as the cohort effect. The cohort effect, by isolating the changes to one segment of the population, helps to predict future rates better than mere extrapolation from the observed changes. The study of the sources of real changes in rates helps one to better understand their causes as well as their consequences for subsequent years.

Questions to Ask in Rating a Rate

The following set of questions to ask in rating a rate is designed to review the areas covered and to provide an outline for use in critiquing a flaw-catching exercise or a real investigation of rates. Like the uniform framework, it is divided into selecting a rate, sampling of rates, standardization of rates, statistical significance of rates, and sources of changes or differences in rates.

1. Selection of Rates
   a. Did the authors appreciate that the risk of occurrence of events is dependent upon the number of individuals at risk as measured by the denominator as well as the number of people affected as measured by the numerator?
   b. Did the authors distinguish between an incidence and a prevalence rate?
2. Sampling of Rates
   a. Was the entire population of interest included in the study or were samples used?
   b. If samples were used, did the authors appreciate the inherent sampling error and estimate its size using a standard error?
   c. If samples were used, was the sampling technique random or representative or was additional variation introduced by the method of sampling?
   d. If samples were used, was the size of the samples adequate or was it likely that a large variation was introduced by the small size of the samples?
3. Standardization of Rates
   a. Was standardization necessary when comparing the rates of occurrence of an event in two different populations?
   b. If standardization was necessary, were the rates standardized for factors that are known to affect outcome so that the rates could be fairly compared?
4. Statistical Significance of Rates
   a. When comparing rates obtained by sampling, was a statistical significance test applied to determine the probability of obtaining differences as great or greater than the one observed if no true difference exists in the larger populations?
   b. Was a distinction made between a statistically significant change or difference and one which is clinically important?

The following flaw-catching exercises are designed to give you practice in applying the principles of rating a rate to simulated research articles. Try to apply the uniform framework and the checklist of questions to evaluate and compare the rates developed in the following hypothetical studies. A sample critique is provided for each exercise.

Exercise No. 1: Testicular Cancer

In order to study what was happening to the rates of testicular cancer as a result of new chemotherapy developed in the 1960s, investigators tried to compare the frequency of testicular cancer in 1960 and 1975. During these years there was a large increase in the number of oncologists who frequently saw testicular cancer patients after the diagnoses were made by urologists. Based on solid information, the investigators assumed that there was no major change between 1960 and 1975 in the effort or the ability to make a diagnosis of testicular cancer.

To accomplish their goal, investigators identified all oncologists practicing in a large city in 1960 and 1975. From the records of these practices, they calculated the total number of testicular cancer patients and the city's rate of testicular cancer in 1960 and 1975. They concluded that the prevalence rate of testicular cancer was 20 per 100,000 in 1960 and 100 per 100,000 in 1975.

The authors could not believe that the prevalence rate of testicular cancer had increased fivefold between 1960 and 1975. Thus, they decided to sample randomly 1% of all U.S. hospital pathology departments and count the diagnoses of testicular cancer made in 1960 and 1975. They found that the rate of testicular cancer was 50 per 100,000 ± 5 in 1960 and 55 per 100,000 ± 6 in 1975.

The authors then drew the following conclusions:

1. The first study showed that the risk of developing testicular cancer was on the increase.
2. The second study also demonstrated an increase even though it was a much smaller increase.
3. By including all the oncologists in a large city, the first study was an inherently better study than the second study that relied on sampling, which is an inherently defective method.

4. The investigators finally concluded that both studies supported the contention that there had been a change for the worse in the prognosis of testicular cancer despite the advent of new chemotherapy.

Critique: Exercise No. 1

Let us look at what was done in each study and then attempt to evaluate the conclusion reached by the investigators.

STUDY NO. 1

Selection of Rates

The first study attempted to measure all patients who were undergoing treatment during 1960 and 1975. It was thus a prevalence study, a study of the frequency of the presence of the condition. The only requirement for inclusion was treatment for testicular cancer during 1960 or 1975. Thus, the first study did not measure the risk or rate of developing testicular cancer but the prevalence rate of treatment for testicular cancer.

Sampling of Rates

This first study did not sample a large population. It attempted to perform a complete evaluation of one large city. Was this method an appropriate and accurate means of discovering all the cases of testicular cancer in the city? The answer would depend on whether all or nearly all testicular cancer patients were seen by the oncologists included in the study. If, and only if, all testicular cancer patients were seen by an oncologist would this method provide a good measure of the prevalence rate of testicular cancer in this city.

Statistical Significance of Differences

Since these rates were not produced by sampling, one does not need to apply statistical significance tests to determine if a difference exists. The data may be used directly. The differences found, however, may be neither real nor important. The existence of real differences depends on showing that the differences were not due to artifactual changes in the way the rates were derived. The importance depends on an interpretation of the cause of the differences.

Source of Differences
In 1960 there were far fewer cancer specialists and there was much less that they could do for testicular cancer patients than in 1975. In 1960 it was likely that urologists performed the surgery and oncologists did not necessarily see every testicular cancer patient. Thus, especially in 1960, it is likely that all testicular cancer patients were not included in the records of oncologists. Therefore, the changes may be artifactual, at least in part, and may reflect the larger number of oncologists in 1975 and the greater probability of their involvement in the care of testicular cancer patients.

STUDY NO. 2
The second study, on the other hand, utilized samples randomly drawn from a large population. It attempted to estimate the incidence rate of diagnoses of new cases of testicular cancer in 1960 and 1975.

Selection of Rates
The hospital pathology records reflect the incidence of diagnosis of testicular cancer. They mostly reflect new cases of testicular cancer, and in general, do not include those who were diagnosed in earlier years and who continued to receive treatment. The incidence rates are a better reflection of risk of developing testicular cancer than the prevalence rate. Incidence rates, however, are not directly affected by changes in treatment that affect the prognosis.

Sampling of Rates and Statistical Significance of the Rates
Since these estimates were derived by randomly sampling the nation's hospitals, they are subject to the inherent errors of sampling. The likely size of these errors is reflected in the standard errors included in the estimates. The range—two standard errors both above and below the sample's value—reflects the larger population's likely rate with 95% accuracy. The range for the 1960 value of 50 per 100,000 ± 5 would be 60 to 40 per 100,000. The range for the 1975 value of 55 per 100,000 ± 6 would be 67 to 43 per 100,000. Thus, it is likely that the difference found between 1960 and 1975 can be explained by the random sampling error alone, without providing evidence of any real change in the incidence rates.

Sources of Differences

Since one would expect that hospital pathology records reflect both equal effort and equal ability to make a diagnosis of testicular cancer in 1960 and 1975, there is much less chance in this study that differences, if they existed, would reflect artifactual changes over time.

With these analyses in mind, let us examine the conclusion drawn by the authors.

1. The first study did not show that the rate of development of testicular cancer was on the increase. As a prevalence study, the first investigation did not even attempt to assess the risk of developing testicular cancer. An incidence study is needed to assess risk. Prevalence rates measure the likelihood of the condition being present at a point in time, not of its developing. Thus, even if the changes can be believed, they do not necessarily reflect increased risk of developing testicular carcinoma. They may reflect the longer survival time of cancer patients due to advances in therapy. As previously noted, however, these changes in the prevalence rate over time may be artifactual because the 1960 rates probably reflect incomplete identification of those with testicular carcinoma.

2. The second study cannot be said to demonstrate a change. Even though the estimates from the second study appeared to increase from 50 to 55 per 100,000 between 1960 and 1975, these differences are well within the inherent sampling error. Thus, no statistically significant difference between the rates exists, and it is likely that the differences are due to chance.

3. The first study was not an inherently better study than the second study. These studies used different methods to measure different rates. The use of sampling is not an inherently inferior method and even may be superior at times to completely studying every individual in one segment of a population. Attempts to study every individual may actually be "chunk sampling," that is, studying only easily available, unrepresentative segments of a large population. The method of random sampling that uses large enough samples is an accurate, time-tested means of producing reliable data. It is not inherently defective.

4. Neither study speaks to the prognosis once testicular cancer has

developed. The first study of oncologists is a prevalence study; it attempts to measure the rate at which testicular cancer was present in a large city in 1960 and 1975. This prevalence rate is indirectly affected by prognosis. If patients are undergoing long-term treatment instead of dying rapidly, then the prevalence rate may increase in the presence of improved prognosis. On the other hand, if patients are rapidly cured and leave treatment, then the prevalence rate may fall in the presence of improved prognosis. The second study is an incidence study. It attempts to measure the rate of development of testicular carcinoma in 1960 and 1975. Changes in the prognosis of testicular cancer cannot be expected to directly affect the rate of its development. Thus, neither study provides evidence for changes in the prognosis as a result of the new chemotherapy. To study changes in prognosis, investigators would need to determine the length of survival of comparable patients diagnosed in 1960 and 1975.

Tuberculosis

An international group of tuberculosis (TB) experts decided to compare the rates of death from TB in the United States to those of India to determine if any lessons could be learned. They knew that TB was quite common in the U.S. before 1950, but that it had declined substantially. They also knew that most individuals who are infected are able to control but not eliminate the infection totally.

Using a large, carefully designed random sampling, the investigators found that the rate of death due to TB in 1975 was 200 per 100,000 ± 10 in India versus 20 per 100,000 ± 5 in the U.S. They also found that the rate for individuals in the 65- to 80 year-old age group was 200 per 100,000 ± 10 in India and 200 per 100,000 ± 10 in the U.S.

Since the investigators knew that India had a much younger population than did the U.S. and that age affects the risk of TB, they tried to age-standardize the rates. They applied the rates for each age group from the U.S. population to the number of individuals in that age group in India. They found that there were 1,000,000 deaths due to TB in India in 1975. They also found that there would have been 50,000 deaths in the U.S. if there had been the same age distribution as in India. The authors drew the following conclusions:

1. The large difference in rates of death between India and the U.S. may have been due to chance.

2. They noted that the rates of death in the U.S. for the 65- to 80-year-old age group is much higher than the average U.S. rate. They concluded that as the average age of the U.S. population gets older, TB will become more of a problem.

3. In comparing the unstandardized rates, it appeared that India had 10 times the U.S. rate of TB. Once standardization was completed, it showed that India had 20 times as much TB. The authors concluded that some mistake must have been made since rate standardization should not make the differences in rates look larger than prestandardized rates. Thus, they concluded that contrasting the overall rates was the fairest means of comparison.

Critique: Exercise No. 2
Selection of Rates
The death rates used in this study of the United States and India are incidence rates of death that are designed to measure the risk of dying from TB in the two countries. Incidence rates of death approximate the risk of death unless the death rates are enormous. Despite the 1,000,000 deaths due to TB in India, this very high rate is still small in comparison to the population of India; therefore the death rate can be used to approximate the risk of death.

Sampling and Statistical Significance
Both the Indian and the American rates purport to be large, carefully designed random samples. As samples, they are estimates of the true rates. The standard errors included with the sample estimates allow one to calculate easily the 95% confidence limits for the rates in each larger population. Thus, the Indian rate of 200 per 100,000 $\pm$ 10 means that the rate for the Indian population is between 220 and 180 per 100,000 with 95% probability. The American rate of 20 per 100,000 $\pm$ 5 means that with 95% probability the U.S. rate is between 10 and 30 per 100,000.

The statistical significance of the differences can be appreciated by looking at those ranges of estimated values for the true population rates. Even if India's true rate is the lower limit of 180 per 100,000, this is far greater than the 30 per 100,000 estimated for the U.S. Thus by understanding the meaning of standard error and calculating the confidence limits of the estimate, it can be seen that the results are statistically significant. One can then reject the null hypothesis of no difference and conclude that the differences in rates between the two countries are likely to be due to more than chance.

Standardization of Rates
The investigators correctly concluded that rate standardization for age was an important procedure if the rates were to be fairly compared. Standardization is important since the populations have a markedly different age distribution, and age is related to the risk of dying from TB. The Indian population is generally younger than the U.S. population. Deaths from TB are concentrated among the old and the very young, thus age standardization is necessary if a fair comparison is to be achieved. The procedure for age standardization was correctly performed. By applying the rates for each age group in the U.S. population to the number of individuals in that age group in the Indian population, the investigators were asking how many deaths there would have been in the U.S. population if there were the same number of individuals in each age group as in India. This number can then be compared directly to the number of deaths that actually occurred in India.

Sources of Differences
Before concluding that these statistically significant differences are real, one must consider whether artifactual differences either in effort or in ability to recognize TB occur between the two countries and whether these factors could explain the differences found. If one assumes that India—with its enormous health problems—is less able than the United States to recognize TB as the cause of death, this fact would actually increase the already large differences found. Thus, artifactual differences in the effort or ability to recognize deaths from TB are not likely to explain or eliminate the differences found.

Assuming that the differences are real, can anything be said about the source and importance of these differences? The authors have noted that the rates among the 65- to 80-year-old age group are identical in the U.S. and in India. This suggests that the U.S. experiences a death rate among the elderly that is much higher than among the rest of the U.S. population, which may be due to some permanent susceptibility among the U.S. elderly. On the other hand, it may reflect a cohort effect. Remember, a cohort effect is a unique, temporary susceptibility among one group or cohort owing to a special past experience. Historically, we know that TB was a much more common disease in the U.S. prior to 1950. In addition, we know that individuals who have been previously infected frequently control the infection but often do not eliminate it totally. These individuals have the possibility of subsequently developing active disease, especially when they become elderly. Thus, it is possible that the high rate among the U.S. elderly is related to their experience in an era when TB was quite frequent. If the cohort effect explains the high TB rate among the U.S. elderly, then it is not likely that the high U.S. rate among those 65 to 80 years old will continue to increase as the proportion of elderly in the U.S. population increases. The rates for this age group may actually fall as less susceptible cohorts advance into this age group.

In India, on the other hand, the rate for the 65- to 80-year-old age group is the same as the general Indian population. Thus, in India, there is no reason to believe that a cohort effect is operating. The rates for all age groups may be uniformly high and the elderly do not necessarily share a unique susceptibility. This implies that if the Indian population experiences an increase in the proportion of elderly, they may not experience much change in the risk of dying from TB.

With this analysis in mind, let us evaluate the conclusions reached by the "experts."

1. It is very unlikely that the differences between the U.S. and India are due to chance. The wide separation of these statistically significant differences makes it most unlikely that chance alone explains the differences. It is never feasible to totally exclude the possibility that chance explains differences found. However, when the values obtained are far outside the confidence limits for the other population, it is standard statistical procedure to reject the null hypothesis of no difference in the larger population. Thus,

by elimination, one accepts the contention that true differences do exist between the U.S. and Indian populations.

2. The fact that the U.S. rates for the 65- to 80-year-old age groups are much higher than the average U.S. rate, does not mean necessarily that TB will become more of a problem as the average age in the U.S. increases. If the high rate for the U.S. elderly is a cohort effect, one would expect a gradual decrease in the rate among the U.S. elderly. This decrease would occur as the younger age groups, who have not lived much of their lives during the times of widespread TB, advance into the 65- to 80-year-old age groups.

3. Standardized rates are a better means of comparing the risk of dying from TB than the overall rates. The standardized rates attempt to adjust for the fact that the two populations have different age distribution. Standardization may make the differences appear smaller or larger. There is no reason to believe that standardization will make big differences look smaller. As illustrated in the factory example during the discussion of standardization (Chap. 21), age-adjustment may even reveal an important difference where none was apparent in the overall rates.

Standardization revealed that the differences between India and the U.S. were even larger than first appreciated. Standardization, however, would have been just as important if the differences afterwards were smaller than first thought. Thus, standardization was properly and appropriately performed in this example.

Selecting a Statistic

PART 4

Introduction and Uniform Framework

To the nonstatistician, the field of statistics at first appears to be composed of a confusing array of tests named from the Greek alphabet. Therefore, if statistics sounds like Greek to you, there is justification for your confusion. There are other sources as well for the nonstatistician's confusion. Good clinicians know the importance of clinical judgment in medicine. Likewise, the good statistician appreciates that good judgment is critical to the proper application of statistics. Unfortunately, the statistically naive can be mesmerized by the mathematics of many medical research articles. This is compounded by the tendency of authors to present data in its most favorable light.

Darrell Huff illustrates the dangers of these dual tendencies. Huff points out that "many a statistic is false on its face. It gets by only because the magic of numbers brings about a suspension of common sense . . ." and that "statistics are as much an art as a science. A great many manipulations and even distortions are possible within the bounds of propriety. Often the statistician must choose among methods, a subjective process, and find the one that he will use to represent the facts." [*How to Lie with Statistics*. New York: Norton, 1954, pp. 120 and 138.] The potential for misleading with statistics, however, should not cause clinicians to downgrade the discipline. Rather it should encourage them to seek a better understanding of statistical methods and their enormous usefulness when correctly applied.

An adequate understanding of statistical methods for an intelligent reader of the medical literature does not require mathematical sophistication. It requires only that the reader have an understanding of what questions statistical equations ask, what choices of methods are available for answering the questions, and what the answers mean. Without an organized approach the reader can be caught in the quicksand of statistics. To help you find your way out of this maze, we will develop a uniform framework for selecting a statistic. Our aim in discussing statistical methods will be to answer the following questions.

1. What question is being asked by the statistical method being used?

2. Is the method appropriate to the type of data being collected?
3. Are the conclusions drawn from the statistical procedure appropriate?

Basic Statistical Methods

The field of statistics may be divided into population statistics and sample statistics. Population statistics, as the name implies, describes populations; these statistics are applied whenever all the individuals who make up the population one wishes to study are included in the investigation. Including the entire population has an advantage in that the differences found can be assumed to be true differences, and the rates observed can be assumed to be true rates since the conclusions are not based on partial samples of the population. Thus, in population statistics one merely needs to measure the associations or differences found and report them. Statistical significance tests are not necessary since statistical significance tests are designed to measure the probability of obtaining the observed results in samples, if no true difference or association exists in the larger populations. When entire populations are actually used, there is no sampling error and no need for statistical significance tests.

Census data and death certificate data are examples of efforts to include the entire population. When United States death rates from breast cancer are reported, for example, these are not estimates, they are actual rates. When the differences in death rates between states are reported, they too are actual differences because they aim to include everyone who died. There is no need to apply statistical significance tests when all individuals who could be included are actually included.

Unfortunately, it is usually impractical or impossible to include the entire population one would like to study. If there are 20 million hypertensives or 1 million individuals with ulcers in the United States, it usually is impossible to include them all in a study; therefore most medical studies are based only on samples of a particular population. The field of sample statistics makes up most of the field of statistics. In fact, statisticians refer to the characteristic of a sample as a "statistic" in order to distinguish a sample characteristic from the characteristic of the entire population, which is known by statisticians as a "parameter."

The field of sample statistics rests on the fundamental assumption that the samples drawn from the larger populations are obtained randomly. That is, both the study group and the control group samples are representative of all those in the larger population who could have been included in the study. Remember that statistical significance tests require random samples, but not randomization between study and control groups. If this assumption of random samples is not true, the results obtained in the study cannot be directly or reliably extrapolated to the larger population. This does not mean that statistical methods can be used only for samples that are randomly obtained from larger populations. It does imply however that the statistical results from a study using nonrandom samples cannot be extrapolated directly to the larger population. If nonrandom samples are used, clinical judgement must be employed in conjunction with statistical analysis when extrapolating from study data to individuals not included in the study.

To organize the use of sample statistics as applied to medical studies, it will help to distinguish two situations in which statistical techniques are commonly used.

1. Investigators are frequently interested in measuring the difference in outcome between groups. They may want to measure the difference in the white blood cell count between black people and white people or the difference in the proportion of men and women with a positive skin test for tuberculosis.

2. Statistical techniques are often used in the study of associations. An association implies that two or more measurements are made on the same individuals. For instance, investigators may want to study the relationship between high blood pressure, high cholesterol, and myocardial infarction or the relationship between height and weight.

The uniform framework outlined in Figure 26-1 begins by distinguishing between the statistical methods used for entire populations and the statistical methods used for samples. Remember that the methods used when the entire population is included in a study are the same as the methods used for sample statistics, except that no statistical significance tests are necessary.

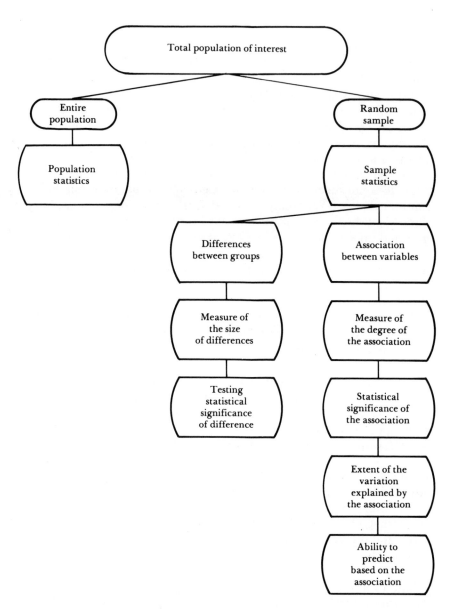

FIGURE 26-1. Uniform framework for the use of statistical methods.

The uniform framework then distinguishes between differences and associations. In studying differences, the interest is in measuring the size of the difference between groups and testing the statistical significance of any differences that are found.

When associations are considered, again the interest is in a measure of the strength or degree of association as well as whether a statistically significant association is present. In studying associations, however, there are two additional considerations that must be addressed: how much of the variation in outcome between individuals is explained by the association being studied, and how useful the association under study is in predicting outcomes for individuals not included in a study.

Types of Data

In organizing our approach to statistical methods, we will distinguish three different types of data: nominal, ordinal, and continuous. The distinction between nominal, ordinal and continuous data is crucial to any approach to statistical methods since the type of data used largely determines the general type of statistical techniques that are applicable.

Nominal data implies that a piece of datum fits into one of a limited number of categories, but the categories cannot be ordered one above another. For instance, the category for race can be white, black, or oriental, and the category for hair color can be blond, brunette or red. Despite the existence of more than two categories, it is not possible to order one above the other. Thus nominal data means that the categories can be named but not ordered.

Ordinal data describes a limited number of categories that can be ordered one above another, but this does not mean that the space between each category is the same. Cancer, for example, may be categorized in stages 1 through 4, and heart disease may be categorized by functional class. There is an inherent ordering of these stages or classes, although the distance between any two stages or classes may not be the same. Ordinal data thus implies that the data can be ordered.

Continuous data states that there are an unlimited number of equally spaced categories; thus a continuum of values is possible. Height and weight are examples of continuous data. A person can weight 100.5 lbs, 101 lbs, 101.1 lbs or an infinite number of points in between. The difference between 100 and 101 lbs is the same as the difference between 105 and 106 lbs. Notice that continuous data does not imply that there is unlimited variation among human beings.

Having distinguished between sample and population statistics, between difference and associations, and between the three different types of data, we will now proceed to take up each of the remaining items in the uniform framework.

In studying the differences between groups, important statistical questions are: What is the size of the difference observed in the data? Are the differences statistically significant? The size of the difference is a measure obtained directly from nominal, ordinal, and continuous data that attempts to compare the outcome in one group versus the outcome in another group. In contrast, the question of statistical significance attempts to relate the observed data to the true values in the parent populations from which the study subjects were obtained. Therefore, the question of the size of the difference quantitates the observed difference, while statistical significance testing asks whether the observed difference is likely to reflect a true difference in the larger populations.

Assessing the Size of Differences

The measure of the differences between groups whose data is nominal or ordinal is a simple measure of the size of the difference. The *size of the difference* is merely the difference between the proportion of individuals with a particular outcome in each group. For instance, if Group A has a 30% cure rate and Group B has a 20% cure rate, the difference between Group A and Group B is 10%.

However, the differences between groups where data consists of continuous measurement cannot be expressed by one simple measure. Figure 27-1 describes the differences between two groups whose data consist of a continuous measurement, in this case the weights of a sample group of males and a sample group of females.

It should be clear from the curves in Figure 27-1 that there is no simple, all-inclusive measure of the difference between the two groups. In describing these differences, statisticians use two types of measure. The first measure, the *mean* or *average* value, is the most commonly used measure of the central point of the data: It is the sum of all observations divided by the number of observations. When calculating the difference between groups, one begins by calculating the difference between the mean values of the groups. The second measure, the *standard deviation*, describes the dispersion, spread, or variation within data for each sample. Math-

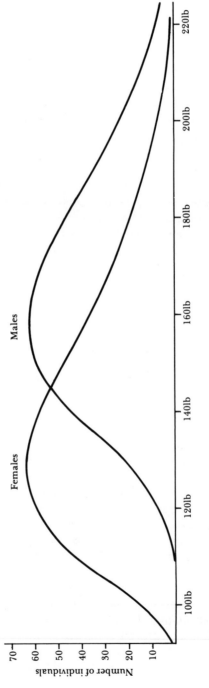

FIGURE 27-1. Possible distribution of the weights of males and females in the same general population.

ematically, the standard deviation takes into account the distance of each point from the mean value of the group.

In order to better understand the need for a measure of the spread of the data within each group, Figure 27-2 illustrates the important principle that curves with equal differences between means can have very different relationships. In the first graph the curve shows no overlap while considerable overlap exists in the second graph.

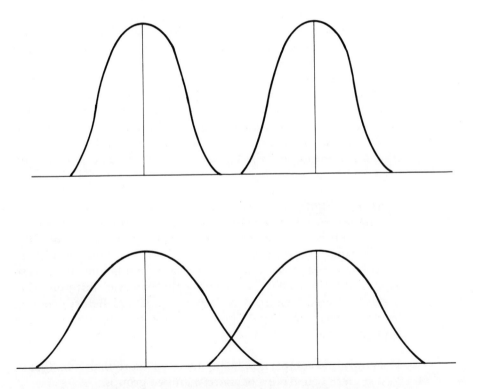

FIGURE 27-2. Distributions with identical differences between their mean or average value but with different degrees of overlap.

The measure called standard deviation allows one to better understand the spread of the data within each group and the degree of the overlap between groups. When the data from each group follows a normal or *Gaussian distribution,* then 95% of each group's measurements are found within two standard deviations above and below the group's mean value. Thus it is important to know when a group's values are normally distributed. Among the features of this distribution are the following characteristics:

1. Continuous symmetrical distribution
2. A mean that lies at the highest point on the curve
3. A shape that approximates a bell-shaped curve

Many measurements on human populations do not follow this distribution. However, statisticians have shown that—regardless of the distribution of the data—at least 75% of all values will lie within two standard deviations of the average and that at least 88% will lie within three standard deviations. Therefore, despite the shape of the data from each group, standard deviations used in conjunction with the means from each group will give an idea of the spread of the data within each group and the degree of the overlap between groups. When examining the differences between groups where the measurement is continuous, one should look at the differences in means as well as the standard deviation of each group.

Statistical Significance of Differences
Having measured the size of the differences observed in the data, one is ready to address the question of statistical significance. Remember that a statistical significance test asks the question: If there is no true difference between the larger populations of interest, what is the probability of obtaining the observed difference between samples drawn from the larger population? Before choosing to use a specific statistical significance test, investigators must answer three basic questions.

1. Is only one comparison being made, or more than one, that is, are there two groups or more than two groups?
2. Have the study and control group individuals been matched (paired)?

3. Will a one-tailed or a two-tailed statistical significance test be used?

The selection of a proper statistical significance test depends upon the answers to these questions as well as upon the type of data (nominal, ordinal, or continuous) being used in a study.

COMPARISONS

The number of comparisons that can be made in a study depends on the number of groups being compared. When there are only two groups, for instance, one study and one control group, then only one comparison is possible. The choice of a statistical significance test depends on whether there is one comparison being made or more than one. When more than one comparison is possible (i.e., three or more groups) the investigator, using all the data, must choose a statistical significance test that is designed to determine whether an overall statistically significant difference is present. Only after determining that such a difference exists, is it legitimate to compare individual groups. Such comparisons of one group to another are known as *pair-wise comparisons.*

To appreciate the need to initially establish an overall statistically significant difference before making pair-wise comparisons, let us look at how the possible comparisons increase as the number of groups increases. For instance, when there are three groups A, B, C, one can make three comparisons: A to B, A to C, and B to C. When there are four groups, A, B, C, D, one can make six comparisons: A to B, A to C, A to D, B to C, B to D, and C to D. As the number of groups increases, the number of comparisons goes up dramatically. Therefore, if individual group comparisons are made when large numbers of groups are involved, chance alone favors finding at least one statistically significant difference. The following rule of thumb demonstrates the danger in making pair-wise comparisons before establishing an overall statistically significant difference.

If a statistically significant difference (p is less than or equal to .05) is incorrectly established by first making all possible pair-wise comparisons, then the true p value equals the observed p value times the number of possible comparisons. For example, if there are four groups and all possible pair-wise comparisons have been made and only group A versus group D reaches statistical significance, then the true p value is calculated as follows:

True p value for
group A versus group D = Observed p value × number
                         of possible comparisons
True p value for
group A versus group D = .05 × 6 = .30

As demonstrated, there is a 30% probability of obtaining the observed difference between one comparison such as group A and group D even if no true difference exists between these groups in the larger population of interest. Statistical tests for pair-wise comparisons are employed after first establishing an overall statistically significant difference. These tests are modifications of the tests that are used when only one comparison is possible; they are modified to make it more difficult to obtain statistically significant p values for individual, pair-wise comparisons. They take into account the fact that chance favors finding a statistically significant difference if enough pair-wise comparisons are made.

MATCHING (PAIRING)
The next consideration in choosing a test is to determine whether the individuals in the study group and the control group are matched or paired. As previously discussed, investigators frequently match or pair study and control individuals to intentionally make the groups more uniform. Individuals in the study and control groups may be paired for age, sex or race if these factors are known to strongly affect the outcome of the study. Investigators may use individuals as a study group and later use the same group as a control group as, for example, when comparing the effects both of a placebo and a new drug on the same individuals' blood pressure.

Matching, when properly used, reduces the number of individuals who are required to demonstrate a statistically significant difference. In statistical language, the ability to detect a statistically significant difference in samples when a true difference exists in the larger population is known as the *statistical power* of the test. Matching or pairing therefore may increase the statistical power of a study. Pairing is actually a special type of matching in which each individual in the study group is compared to one particular individual or pair in the control group. When pairing occurs, special statistical methods are necessary in the analysis to take advantage of this type of comparison. Subsequently, when we refer to matching, we will mean that special type of matching technically known as pairing.

ONE-TAILED AND TWO-TAILED TESTS

The final basic consideration in deciding which test to use is to determine whether a one-tailed or a two-tailed test is applicable. To understand what this consideration implies, let us return again to the question being asked by a statistical significance test. A statistical significance test asks what the probability is of obtaining data as extreme or more extreme than the observed data if the null hypothesis is true. Data as extreme or more extreme than that observed may occur in the direction observed or it may occur in the opposite direction. For instance if sample group A has an average value of 30 and sample group B has an average value of 25, then the difference in averages between group A and group B is 5. A *two-tailed significance test* asks the question: What is the probability of obtaining a difference of five or more between group A and group B in either direction if the null hypothesis were true? In other words, if no true difference exists in the larger population and group A averages 30, what is the probability that group B's average will be ≤ 25 or ≥ 35? A *one-tailed test* asks only what the probability is that a difference as great or greater would occur in the direction observed. Thus, a one-tailed test asks the question: If no true difference exists in the larger population and group A's average is 30, what is the probability that group B's average will be ≤ 25?

The decision whether to use a one-tailed or two-tailed test is a clinical decision and not a statistical one; it depends on the study question being asked. A two-tailed test is appropriate when there is interest in differences in the opposite direction. For instance, if one hypothesized that a new therapy increased the chances of survival over those of the standard treatment, one would also be interested in results that showed the new treatment to be worse than the standard treatment.

A one-tailed test is appropriate if the interest is only in the results in one direction. If a difference has been well established already, the size of the difference might be studied. For instance, one might hypothesize that on the average American women live three years longer than American men. If the data collected indicated that in the study sample men live longer than women, the results could be attributed to an unusual sample and there would be no interest in data in the opposite direction.

Therefore the reader and investigator must ask: Would one be interested in the results if they occurred in the opposite direction from the hypothesis? When in doubt it is preferable to use two-tailed tests. The two-tailed test has less statistical power, but more faith can be placed in a statistically significant result obtained using a two-tailed test rather than a one-tailed test. The burden of proof is on the investigator who uses a one-tailed test rather than a two-tailed one.

Specific Tests for Specific Data

Having discussed the three important distinctions to make regardless of the type of data, let us turn our attention to the specific tests to choose for nominal, ordinal, and continuous data.

NOMINAL DATA: CHI SQUARE METHODS

Chi Square methods are the most commonly used techniques for nominal data. They can be used for one comparison or modified for more than one comparison.

It is important to know when the numbers are large enough to use a Chi Square test, which requires an understanding of how a Chi Square test is performed. The Chi Square statistic is calculated by creating a box chart and predicting how many individuals would be in each box if the null hypothesis were true. For instance, if researchers were studying the difference in the five-year survival rate of 50 patients in group 1 given a new cancer treatment and 50 patients in group 2 given the standard treatment, the results might be as follows:

	GROUP 1	GROUP 2	
Survivors	40	6	46
Deaths	10	44	54
	50	50	100

To determine if the Chi Square technique is appropriate, one needs to calculate from this data the numbers in each box that would be expected if the null hypothesis of no difference in treatment were true. If 46 patients are known to survive at five years and if the treatment makes no difference, 50% of them would be in group 1 and 50% in group 2. Thus 23 people are expected to survive in each group if the null hypothesis holds true. Similarly, if 54 are known to be dead before 5 years and the null hypothesis were true, then there would be 27 dead in group 1 and 27 dead in group 2. The expected numbers can be expressed as follows:

	GROUP 1	GROUP 2	
Survivors	23	23	46
Deaths	27	27	54
	50	50	100

Notice that in our example we used 50 patients in each group. This means that one could expect 50% of the dead and 50% of the living to come from each population. Parallel methods exist for calculating expected numbers when the sizes of the groups are unequal.

In applying Chi Square methods, the expected numbers are compared to the observed numbers. However, Chi Square methods should not be used when the expected numbers are very small. In general, if the expected number in any box is less than five, the Chi Square technique should not be used. In such cases a test known as Fischer's exact test is applicable but quite laborious, especially as the sizes of the groups increase. Fischer's test is useful only when two groups are being compared. Since the expected numbers are 23 or 27 in our examples, the Chi Square would be appropriate. When the Chi Square method is used for comparing two groups, there is a special modification known as Yates Correction for continuity, which generally should be used.

The test for nominal data with matched samples is a modification of the Chi Square method known as McNemar's test. Except for its use with matched samples, its applicability is parallel with the Chi Square test. When matched study samples are too small to use

McNemar's test, a test known as the sign test can be used. One-and two-tailed modifications of these tests are available. Table 27-1 summarizes the use of statistics to study differences between groups whose data are nominal.

ORDINAL DATA: NONPARAMETRIC TESTS
Ordinal data can fall into many categories, but there is not necessarily an equal distance between the categories. A class of statistical significance tests known as nonparametric tests is suited uniquely to ordinal data. Nonparametric methods are applicable to very small groups so that one is rarely concerned with choosing the appropriate test on the basis of sample size.

Nonparametric tests have not been used widely in medical studies, which is unfortunate because they are very useful tests. The tests can be used whenever data can be ordered or ranked regardless of how many categories are present or how distant the categories are from one another. Therefore, when it is not clear that data are really continuous, it is best to combine the data into discrete, ordered categories, that is, make the data ordinal and use nonparametric methods. There is some loss of statistical power when using nonparametric techniques compared to parametric tests used for continuous data, but the loss is often surprisingly small.

In choosing an appropriate statistical significance test for ordinal data, the same basic questions are asked: 1) How many comparisons are being made? 2) Have the study and control group individuals

TABLE 27-1. STATISTICAL PROCEDURES FOR DIFFERENCES WITH NOMINAL DATA

Type of study samples	Tests of the statistical significance of the difference
Small, unmatched sample, 1 comparison	Fischer's exact test
Small, matched sample, 1 comparison	Sign test
Large, unmatched sample, 1 or more comparisons	Chi Square
Large, matched sample, 1 or more comparisons	McNemar's test

been matched? 3) Is one interested in a one-tailed or a two-tailed comparison? When making only one comparison where the study groups are not matched, the Mann-Whitney U test or the median test is applicable. When making one comparison where the study groups are matched, the Wilcoxon matched-pairs signed-ranks test is the appropriate test. When more than one comparison is being made and the groups are not matched, the Kruskal-Wallis 1-way analysis of variance is used. Finally, when there is more than one comparison and the groups are matched, the Friedman 2-way analysis of variance method is appropriate. One- and two-tailed modifications are available for each test. Table 27-2 summarizes the choice of statistical significance tests for ordinal data.

CONTINUOUS DATA: t TEST AND F TEST
The considerations in choosing an appropriate test for continuous data are the same as for ordinal data. The first consideration is to determine how many study groups are being compared and whether the groups are matched. For one comparison with unmatched groups, the proper test is known as the *t test,* which is sometimes referred to as the *student t test.* When more than one comparison is being made, the proper test for continuous data is known as the *F test.* With more than one comparison, the F test should be applied first to establish that a statistically significant difference exists somewhere in the data. Having established the existence of an overall, statistically significant F test, one can apply a modification of the t test known as the Scheffe test to determine

TABLE 27-2.   STATISTICAL PROCEDURES USED WITH ORDINAL DATA

	Type of study samples	Tests of the statistical significance of the difference
One comparison (two groups)	Unmatched sample	Mann-Whitney U or median test
	Matched sample	Wilcoxon matched-pairs signed-ranks test
More than one comparison (more than two groups)	Unmatched sample	Kruskal-Wallis 1-way analysis of variance
	Matched sample	Friedman 2-way analysis of variance

which comparison or comparisons make contributions to the overall difference.

When the data are matched, modifications of both the F and the t tests are available. The t test for matched samples is used for studying the differences between two groups. The modification of the F test for matched groups is known as the F test for analysis of variance with blocking; an alternate known as analysis of covariance may also be used.

One- and two-tailed modifications of t tests are also available. Again, the two-tailed version is used unless there is a strong reason to do otherwise. Table 27-3 summarizes the statistical significance tests used for continuous data.

When confronted with continuous data from two groups presented as mean values plus and minus a standard deviation, it is often very helpful to rapidly calculate your own t test. Fortunately, when the sample size of each group is larger than 30, a few relatively simple calculations allow one to perform an approximate t test. In the process of making these calculations it is possible to get a better appreciation of the relationship between the spread of the data of the individual sample and the existence of a statistically significant difference.

This conversion utilizes the concept of confidence limits, particularly, the 95% confidence limits that estimate with 95% reliability the range within which the larger population's average lies. The

TABLE 27-3. STATISTICAL PROCEDURES FOR DIFFERENCES WITH CONTINUOUS DATA

	Types of study samples	Tests of the statistical significance of the difference
One comparison (two groups)	Unmatched sample	t test
	Matched sample	
		Matched t test
More than one comparison (more than two groups)	Unmatched sample	F test for analysis of variance
	Matched sample	
		F test for analysis of variance with blocking or analysis of covariance

calculation of the 95% confidence limits requires three pieces of data: the sample's standard deviation, the sample's size, and the sample's mean. All three pieces of information generally are available in any study that is written up for publication.

The creation of the 95% confidence limits requires that we calculate the measure known as the standard error of the mean. The standard error of the mean has the following relationship to standard deviation and sample size:

$$\text{Standard error of the mean} = \frac{\text{Standard deviation}}{\sqrt{\text{Sample size}}}$$
(i.e., number of individuals in the group)

The standard error of the mean is a measure of how close the sample's average is to our best estimate of the larger population's average. This best estimate of the larger population's average is expressed by the 95% confidence limit that utilizes the standard error of the mean as follows:

$$95\% \text{ confidence limit} = \text{Sample's average} \pm 2 \times \text{Standard error of the mean}$$

Suppose the average weight in pounds of 400 boys, 10 years old, was presented as 100 ± 16 with 100 representing the average weight and 16 representing the standard deviation. To calculate the estimate of the average weight of the larger population from which these boys were sampled, it is necessary to calculate the 95% confidence limits as follows:

$$\text{Standard error of the mean} = \frac{\text{Standard deviation}}{\sqrt{\text{Sample size}}} = \frac{16}{\sqrt{400}} = \frac{16}{20} = .8$$

Thus the 95% confidence limits:

$$\text{Sample average} \pm 2 \times \text{Standard error of the mean} =$$
$$100 \pm 2 \times .8 = 100 \pm 1.6$$

Therefore the 95% confidence limits equal 98.4 to 101.6 pounds, which says that with 95% certainty the average weight of 10-year-old boys in the larger population is between 98.4 and 101.6 pounds.

To compare two samples to determine whether a statistically significant difference exists, it is necessary to calculate the 95%

confidence limits for each sample. Having derived both confidence limits, one then is ready to look at the question of statistical significance. *A statistically significant difference exists if the 95% confidence limit for one sample fails to overlap the average of the other sample.* Notice that it is not a question of the confidence limits overlapping, but whether the confidence limits from one population overlap the sample's average in the other population.

To illustrate this procedure, suppose that a sample of 100 girls, 10 years old, was compared to the previous sample of 10-year-old boys. The sample of girls is found to be 105 pounds ± 20. In other words the average weight of the sample is 105 pounds and the standard deviation is 20.

The standard error of the mean for the girls would be:

$$\text{Standard error of the mean} = \frac{\text{Standard deviation}}{\sqrt{\text{Sample size}}} = \frac{20}{\sqrt{100}} = \frac{20}{10} = 2$$

95% confidence limits = Sample's average ± 2 × Standard error of the mean = 105 ± 2 × 2 = 105 ± 4

Thus the 95% confidence limits range from 101 to 109 pounds.

Having derived the confidence limits for the sample of girls and for the sample of boys, it is possible to look at the statistical significance of this difference. The sample's average for the boys equals 100. The lower limits of the 95% confidence range for the girls is 101. Thus the confidence range of the girl's sample does not overlap the average of the boy's sample. Similarly, the 95% confidence limits of the boys extends to 101.6. This range does not overlap the girl's sample average of 105. It is possible therefore to conclude that a statistically significant difference exists between the weights of the boys and the girls.*

Notice that the confidence limits themselves overlap (i.e., boys 98.4 to 101.6; girls 101 to 109), but that the confidence limits do not overlap the averages from the other sample. Notice also that this example illustrates the fact that relatively small differences can be statistically significant when the number of individuals used to obtain the sample is relatively large.

*In many journal articles, data from samples will be expressed as means plus or minus one standard error instead of one standard deviation. When this occurs, one can calculate the confidence limits directly.

Medical investigations—whether they be retrospective, cross-sectional, prospective or experimental studies—frequently attempt to evaluate associations rather than differences. In medical studies, an association implies that two characteristics occur together more often than would be expected by chance. In studying associations the investigators measure two or more characteristics on the same individual.

For instance, the researcher may be interested in an association between estrogens and endometrial cancer, or high cholesterol, high blood pressure, and myocardial infarction. In many medical studies one of the factors (such as endometrial cancer or myocardial infarction) may be regarded as the outcome while the other factors are studied to determine whether they are risk factors* associated with the outcome. Statisticians refer to these outcomes as dependent variables because they are being examined to see whether the occurrence of these outcomes is dependent on the occurrence of the other factors. In contrast, estrogens, high blood pressure, and high cholesterol would be considered independent variables.

It is important to keep in mind that the existence of an association does not prove a cause and effect relationship; it is merely a starting point in studying cause and effect. Contributory cause not only requires the existence of an association, it also requires that the cause precede the effect and that altering the cause alters the effect.

To help define the questions that one would like to answer in dealing with potential associations, let us imagine that an investigator was studying the relationship between high cholesterol and myocardial infarction. Here, high cholesterol can be considered the independent variable and myocardial infarction can be considered the dependent variable or outcome. In studying this relationship the investigator might proceed as follows.

First the researcher collects sample data using one of the study designs such as a retrospective or prospective study in order to

*The term *risk factor* does not have a consistent meaning. At times it is used to imply an association without any implication that the risk factor precedes the disease. At other times it implies a prior association. In other words, the term *risk factor* may or may not imply that the risk factor fulfills our first criteria for cause and effect, that is, the cause precedes the effect. The term *risk factor* as it will be used in this discussion means the same as *independent variable*, which is associated with a dependent variable without implying that it precedes the dependent variable.

determine the strength or degree of association between high cholesterol and myocardial infarction.

If high cholesterol is found to have a strong association with myocardial infarction, the investigator will ask the question: Is the association found in the sample data statistically significant? In other words, if there is no true association in the larger population, what is the probability of obtaining the observed or greater degree of association in the sample data by chance alone?

If the association is found to be statistically significant, the researcher asks another question: How much of the risk of having a myocardial infarction among those included in the investigation is attributable to high cholesterol? The researcher is asking how much of the variation in the dependent or outcome variable (myocardial infarction) among the study individuals can be explained by the occurrence of the risk factor or independent variable (high cholesterol). Thus investigators who study association desire answers to these three questions:

1. What is the degree or the strength of the association?
2. Is the association found in the sample data statistically significant?
3. How much of the risk of developing the condition is attributable to the risk factor? In other words, how much of the variation in the outcome in the study and control groups is explained by the association?

Nominal Data

Let us apply these general concepts of studying associations to the types of studies discussed earlier. First, we will look at the statistical techniques for nominal data that are useful for prospective and experimental studies. Then we will turn to techniques used in retrospective and cross-sectional studies of association when nominal data are employed.

In developing our approach to associations for prospective and experimental studies with nominal data, let us assume that we are studying the association between birth control pills and thrombophlebitis. We will attempt to assess whether birth control pills are a risk factor in the development of the disease. In this case, the use of birth control pills is the independent variable and thrombophlebitis is the dependant variable. In order to determine whether a characteristic such as the use of birth control pills is a risk factor, we need to assess whether its use increases the risk of developing thrombophlebitis. But first, let us review the concept of risk.

The risk of developing a condition equals the number of individuals who develop the condition divided by the number of individuals who could have developed the condition. In assessing the risk of developing thrombophlebitis, we would divide the number of women on birth control pills who develop thrombophlebitis by the total number of women on birth control pills. This concept of risk is called the *absolute risk*. It reflects the probability of developing thrombophlebitis in association with the use of birth control pills. Absolute risk is important in and of itself; however, it does not assess the risk of developing thrombophlebitis if a women is not on birth control pills.

A further assessment of risk is necessary in order to measure the relative degree of association between thrombophlebitis and birth control pills. This measure is known as *relative risk*. Relative risk measures the risk of thrombophlebitis if birth control pills are used versus the risk if birth control pills are not used. It is defined as follows:

$$\text{Relative risk} = \frac{\substack{\text{Risk of developing} \\ \text{thrombophlebitis if birth control pills are used}}}{\substack{\text{Risk of developing thrombophlebitis if} \\ \text{birth control pills are not used}}}$$

or more generally,

$$\text{Relative risk} = \frac{\text{Risk of the outcome if the risk factor is present}}{\text{Risk of the outcome if the risk factor is absent}}$$

Let us illustrate how the risk and relative risk are calculated using a hypothetical example.

An investigator followed 1,000 randomly chosen young women on birth control pills and 1,000 randomly chosen young women who were nonusers. He found that 30 of the women on birth control pills developed thrombophlebitis over a 10-year period while only three of the nonusers developed thrombophlebitis. He presented his data as follows:

	THROMBOPHLEBITIS	NO THROMBOPHLEBITIS	
Birth control pills	a = 30	b = 970	a + b = 1000
No birth control pills	c = 3	d = 997	c + d = 1000

The risk of developing thrombophlebitis on birth control pills equals the number of women on the pill who develop thrombophlebitis divided by the total number of women on the pill. Thus,

$$\text{Risk of developing thrombophlebitis for women on pill} = \frac{a}{a + b} = \frac{30}{1{,}000} = 3\%$$

Likewise the risk of developing thrombophlebitis for women not on the pill equals the number of women not on the pill who develop thrombophlebitis divided by the total number of women not on the pill. Thus:

$$\text{Risk of developing thrombophlebitis for women not on pill} = \frac{c}{c + d} = \frac{3}{1{,}000} = 0.3\%$$

The relative risk equals the ratio of these two risks, thus,

$$\text{Relative risk} = \frac{a}{a + b} \bigg/ \frac{c}{c + d} = \frac{3\%}{.3\%} = 10$$

A relative risk of 1 implies that use of birth control pills does not increase the risk of thrombophlebitis. This relative risk of 10 implies that for women on the pill, the risk of thrombophlebitis is increased tenfold compared to women not on the pill.

A statistical test is available to answer our second question: Is the association statistically significant? This test is known as the statistical significance of the relative risk. It answers the question: If there is no increased relative risk from the use of birth control pills among young women in the larger population from which our study sample is drawn, what is the probability of obtaining an as large or larger relative risk as the one obtained?

The third question we must address asks: How much of the risk of thrombophlebitis is attributable to birth control pills? *Attributable risk*, like relative risk, does not imply cause and effect. It attempts to answer the question: How much of the difference in outcome between groups can be explained by the use of birth control pills?

In answering this question, one calculates what percentage of the risk of thrombophlebitis would remain if birth control pills were eliminated from the study population. To do this, one subtracts the absolute risk of thrombophlebitis among those not on the pill from the risk to those on the pill to obtain the risk due to the pill. One then looks at this risk due to the pill as a percentage of the total risk to those on the pill. This allows one to calculate the percentage of the risk of thrombophlebitis for those on the pill, which is really attributable to the pill. We can thus express attributable risk as follows:

$$\text{Attributable risk} = \frac{\begin{array}{c}\text{Risk of developing}\\\text{thrombophlebitis}\\\text{for women on pill}\end{array} - \begin{array}{c}\text{Risk of developing}\\\text{thrombophlebitis}\\\text{for women not on pill}\end{array}}{\begin{array}{c}\text{Risk of developing thrombophlebitis for women}\\\text{not on pill}\end{array}}$$

From our data:

$$\frac{3 - .3}{3} = \frac{2.7}{3} = 90\%$$

Thus in our study population, 90% of the risk of thrombophlebitis is attributable to the pill. Attributable risk has answered our third basic question: How much of the variation in outcome (thrombophlebitis) between groups is explained by the independent variable (use of birth control pills) under study?

We have just outlined the methods for answering our three basic

questions for associations composed of nominal data when prospective and experimental studies are employed. Let us turn to
retrospective and cross-sectional studies and again ask our three
basic questions. Remember that retrospective and cross-sectional
studies both begin by identifying individuals who have the disease
or condition under study. In retrospective studies the investigator
attempts to determine whether the potential risk factor was previously present while cross-sectional studies determine if the potential risk factor is currently present. Otherwise the study designs
are identical.

In assessing how to answer our three basic questions about association, let us return to our study of the association between birth
control pills and thrombophlebitis. We will present data from a
hypothetical cross-sectional study performed as follows.

An investigator randomly selected 100 young women with
thrombophlebitis and 100 young women without thrombophlebitis.
She carefully obtained the history of use of birth control pills. She
found that 90 of the 100 women with thrombophlebitis were using
birth control pills at the time they developed thrombophlebitis
versus the use of birth control pills by 45 of the 100 women without
thrombophlebitis. She represented her data as follows:

	THROMBOPHLEBITIS	NO THROMBO-PHLEBITIS
Birth control pills	a = 90	b = 45
No birth control pills	c = 10	d = 55
	100	100

Notice that in retrospective and cross-sectional studies the investigator has chosen the total number of patients in each group both with and without thrombophlebitis. She could have chosen to select 200 patients with thrombophlebitis and 100 patients without thrombophlebitis or a number of other combinations. Thus the actual numbers in each vertical column can be altered at will by the investigator. In other words, in a retrospective or cross-sectional study the number of individuals who have and do not have the disease does not reflect the natural incidence. It is therefore improper to add the boxes horizontally in a retrospective or cross-sectional study as we did in the prospective study.

Unfortunately, without numbers in the far right-hand side of the figure, it is not possible to calculate absolute risks or relative risks as can be done for prospective and experimental studies. But a good approximation of relative risk exists for these studies, which turns out to be very useful for statistical analysis. This approximation of relative risk is known as the odds ratio. The *odds ratio* measures the odds of having the risk factor if the condition is present divided by the odds of having the risk factor if the condition is not present.

The odds of being on the pill for women with thrombophlebitis is calculated by taking the number of women who develop thrombophlebitis and are on the pill divided by the number of women who develop thrombophlebitis and are not on the pill, thus,

$$\text{Odds of being on pill for women with thrombophlebitis} = \frac{a}{c} = \frac{90}{10} = 9:1$$

Likewise, the odds of being on the pill for women who do not develop thrombophlebitis is measured by taking the number of women who do not have thrombophlebitis and are using the pill divided by the number of women who do not develop thrombophlebitis and are not on the pill, thus,

$$\text{Odds of being on pill if no thrombophlebitis is present} = \frac{b}{d} = \frac{45}{55} = .82:1$$

Parallel with the calculation of relative risk, one can develop a measure of the relative odds of being on the pill if thrombophlebitis is present versus being on the pill if thrombophlebitis is not present. This measure of the strength of association is known as the odds ratio. Thus,

$$\text{Odds ratio} = \frac{\text{Odds of being on pill if thrombophlebitis is present}}{\text{Odds of being on pill if thrombophlebitis is not present}}$$

$$\text{Odds ratio} = \frac{\dfrac{a}{c}}{\dfrac{b}{d}} = \frac{ad}{cb} = \frac{9}{.82} = 11$$

An odds ratio of 1 means that there are no increased odds of being on the pill if thrombophlebitis is present compared to the odds of being on the pill if thrombophlebitis is absent. Our odds ratio of 11 means that the odds of being on birth control pills is increased elevenfold for women with thrombophlebitis. The odds ratio serves as the basic measure of the degree of association for retrospective and cross-sectional studies. It is in and of itself a useful and valid measure of the strength of the association. In addition, as long as the risk factor (use of birth control pills) is not extremely frequent, the odds ratio approximates the relative risk.

It is possible to look at the odds ratio in reverse and come up with the same result. For instance,

$$\text{Odds ratio} = \frac{\text{Odds of developing thrombophlebitis if pill is used}}{\text{Odds of developing thrombophlebitis if pill is not used}}$$

The odds ratio then equals,

$$\frac{\dfrac{a}{b}}{\dfrac{c}{d}} = \frac{ad}{cb}$$

Notice that this is the same formula as the one shown above. This convenient property allows one to calculate an odds ratio from a prospective or experimental study instead of using the relative risk, and compare it directly to the odds ratio produced by a cross-sectional or retrospective study.

Clinically, one can think of the odds ratio as the individual's risk of disease if exposed to a specific factor compared to the risk of disease if not exposed. For instance, if the odds ratio for estrogen and endometrial cancer is 5, then the average women will have five times the risk of developing endometrial cancer if she uses estrogens compared to her risk if she does not use estrogens. In addition, it is possible to perform a statistical significance test on the odds ratio.

We have now approached questions of the strength and statistical significance of association in retrospective and cross-sectional studies using nominal data. Parallel with our discussion of prospective and experimental studies, we need to present a measure of the extent to which the variation in outcome is explained by the risk factor.

In retrospective and cross-sectional studies, it is possible to calculate an approximate attributable risk if one is able to estimate separately the prevalence of the risk factor in the population of interest. In other words, if one wants to determine the extent that thrombophlebitis is attributable to birth control pills among female college students, one must estimate the proportion of female college students who use birth control pills. One then uses this estimate in conjunction with a retrospective or cross-sectional study to calculate the percentage of the risk of thrombophlebitis among female college students that is attributable to birth control pills. Thus, the three basic questions about association can be answered for experimental, prospective, retrospective and cross-sectional studies. Table 28-1 outlines the measures that are used to answer each question.

Ordinal and Continuous Data

Having examined the use of statistical techniques for studying associations employing nominal data, let us look at techniques for studying associations using ordinal or continuous data. As with nominal data, we will be interested in describing the degree or strength of the association, the statistical significance of the association, and the extent to which the variation in one variable can be explained by the other. With ordinal or continuous data, the techniques are the same for all four types of study designs.

The fundamental techniques used to study associations when the data consist of ordinal or continuous measurements is known as correlation. A widely used and important type of correlation technique is known as Pearson's correlation methods. Pearson's methods are useful when both of the following conditions are met.

TABLE 28-1. MEASURES USED TO ANSWER THE THREE BASIC QUESTIONS ABOUT ASSOCIATION WITH NOMINAL DATA

	Degree of association	Statistical significance of association	Extent of variation attributed to the risk factor
Prospective or experimental studies	Relative risk	Statistical significance of the relative risk	Attributable risk from the study data
Retrospective or cross-sectional studies	Odds ratio	Statistical significance of the odds ratio	Attributable risk from the study data plus an estimate of the prevalence of the risk factor in the population of interest

1. Both measurements being correlated consist of continuous data.
2. A linear relationship exists between the variables being correlated.

To better understand the meaning of a linear relationship, let us look at the data in Figure 28-1 that reflect a positive linear correlation between calories consumed and weight for adults. It indicates that as the calories consumed go up so does the weight. The line reflects the best straight line that can be drawn, indicating the linear nature of the relationship. However, a correlation is not always positive. Negative linear correlations may exist as shown in Figure 28-2, reflecting the *decrease* with age in the rate of healing.

In order to determine when Pearson's correlation techniques are appropriate, it is necessary to graph the observed data and determine whether a linear relationship appears to exist. When either variable consists of ordinal data or when a linear relationship does not appear to exist, alternative techniques known as nonparametric correlation methods can be applied.

Pearson's Correlation Techniques

Pearson's product moment correlation is the basic correlation technique for measuring associations when the data from both groups

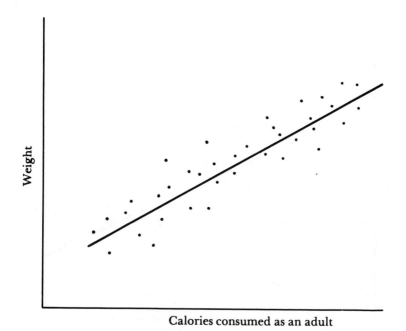

FIGURE 28-1. Example of a positive linear correlation between weight and calories consumed as an adult.

are continuous and a linear relationship is suspected. The degree of association is measured by Pearson's correlation coefficient, which is called r. The value of r can vary from -1 to $+1$. A value of $+1$ implies that a perfect positive correlation exists; a value of -1 implies a perfect negative correlation, and a value of zero implies that change in one variable will have no predictable effect on the other variable.

Let us imagine that we are asking how well systolic blood pressure correlates with diastolic blood pressure. Assume we have applied Pearson's techniques and derived a value of $r = 0.8$. It is now possible to determine whether this value is statistically significant. Here one is asking what the probability is of obtaining an r of 0.8 or greater in either direction if there is no true association in the general population from which the sample data were drawn.

Correlation techniques have a further characteristic that allows one to answer directly our third question, that is, to what extent the variation in diastolic blood pressure explains the variation in systolic blood pressure. If one multiplies r by itself and thus cal-

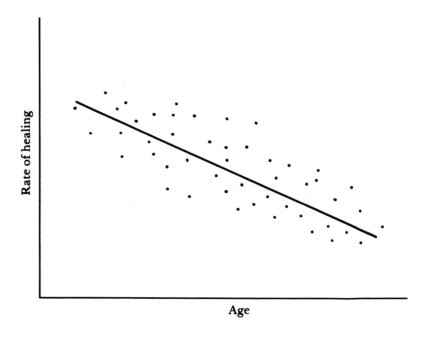

FIGURE 28-2. Example of a negative linear correlation between rate of healing and age.

culates r^2, a new measure called Pearson's coefficient of determination is derived.

In the example, if $r = 0.8$ then $r^2 = 0.64$. Pearson's coefficient of determination has the important characteristic of measuring the extent to which the variation in one measurement is explained by changes in the other. In other words, it measures how much of the variation in the systolic blood pressure is explained by variation in the diastolic blood pressure. Thus in the example, 64% of the variation in systolic blood pressure could be explained by variation in the diastolic blood pressure.

Pearson's correlation techniques can be expanded for more than one comparison. For instance, imagine if one were studying the additional correlation between salt intake, weight, and systolic blood pressure. When Pearson's correlation techniques are used for more than two variables, they are known as multiple correlation and the letter R replaces r. The Rs can be interpreted as the correlation between any two variables with the other variables held

TABLE 28-2. STATISTICAL PROCEDURES USED FOR STUDYING ASSOCIATIONS

	Measure of degree of association	Testing for statistical significance of association	Extent association explains variation between groups
Nominal data	Odds ratio or relative risk	Statistical significance of odds ratio or relative risk	Attributable risk
Continuous data and linear relationship suspected	Pearson's correlation coefficients (r)	Statistical significance of r	r^2
Ordinal data or no linear relationship suspected	Spearman's rho (ρ) or Kendall's tau (τ)	Statistical significance of rho (ρ) or tau (τ)	$rho^2(\rho^2)$ or tau^2 (τ^2)

constant. R^2 then tells us the percentage of the variation in one variable that can be attributed to a second variable if the other study factors are held constant. In our example, an R and R^2 would be calculated for the correlation between salt intake and systolic blood pressure with weight and diastolic blood pressure held constant. Another R and R^2 would be calculated for the correlation between weight and systolic blood pressure with salt intake and diastolic blood pressure held constant.

Nonparametric Correlation
When the data from any of the variables is ordinal or when a linear relationship is not suspected, nonparametric techniques are available that are nearly as statistically powerful as Pearson's correlation coefficients. The two most commonly used nonparametric methods for measuring the degree of correlation are Spearman's rho (ρ) and Kendall's tau (τ). Spearman's rho and Kendall's tau have similar interpretations. They both measure the degree of association, and both have their own statistical significance tests. In addition, as with Pearson's r, both rho and tau can be squared to give a

measure of the extent to which the variation in one variable can be explained by variation in the other.

Kendall's methods can be expanded to deal with more than two variables. Like Pearson's techniques, the results give the percentage of the variation in one variable that can be attributed to a second variable if the other study factors are held constant. Table 28-2 summarizes the ways in which the three basic questions about association can be addressed for nominal, continuous, and ordinal data.

Regression methods represent a series of statistical techniques that are useful for studying the association between one dependent variable and many independent variables. These techniques are capable of measuring the strength of an association, the statistical significance of an association, and the extent of the variation in the dependent variable that can be explained by the independent variable. Thus regression techniques are capable of addressing the first three basic questions about associations.

Regression techniques have two further advantages. First, they allow the study of many associations simultaneously. They serve as techniques for performing multiple simultaneous adjustments by allowing the observer to look at the effect of one independent variable on the dependent variables while the effects of the other independent variables are held constant. Secondly, regression techniques allow the development of a model to see how well the associations under study are able to predict the outcome for individuals not included in the study.

Our discussion of regression methods will cover the following points: how regression methods help to answer the three basic questions about associations; how regression methods allow many independent variables to be taken into account or adjusted for simultaneously; how regression methods can be used to predict an outcome for individuals not included in the study.

We will begin by looking at the relationship between weight and average calories consumed, using a regression technique known as *linear regression* (Fig. 29-1). Linear regression can be used whenever the dependent variable is composed of continuous data—such as weight, for example.

The straight line represents the best line that can be drawn through the data. From this data it is possible to derive a summary expression of the relationship by calculating the slope of the best line that can be drawn through the data.

$$B = \frac{Y}{X} = \frac{\text{Change in the dependent variable}}{\text{Change in the independent variable}}$$

In the example of weight and calories, let us imagine that $X = 100$ and $Y = 10$. Thus,

$$B = \frac{Y}{X} = \frac{10}{100} = .10$$

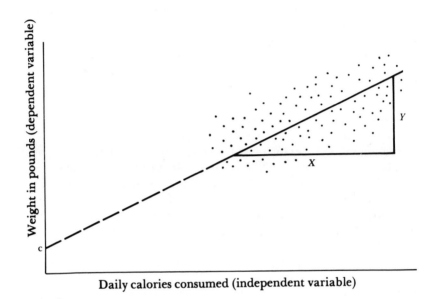

FIGURE 29-1. The association between weight and calories consumed diagrammed for a study using linear regression.

The value of B tells us the strength of the association between calories consumed and weight. Therefore, the average for the range of our data is a 10-pound increase in weight for every increase of 100 calories in daily consumption. Thus B answers our first basic question: How strong is the association?

Regression methods attempt to construct equations that describe the nature of the relationship being studied. For this simple case of a linear or straight line relationship involving one dependent and one independent variable, the regression line would be expressed as follows:

$Y = BX + c$

Y = current weight

X = current daily calories consumed

B = the slope of the best straight line that can be drawn through the data

c = a constant reflecting the value of Y if the straight line is extended to the point where $X = 0$.

A statistical significance test can be performed on B. The statistical significance test asks: If there is no predictable change in Y (weight) for each change in X (daily calories consumed) in the larger population, what is the probability of obtaining sample data with a value of B as great or greater than the one obtained? Thus the statistical significance of B addresses our second basic question concerning associations.

Finally, there are methods that are available in regression for asking how much of the variation in Y (weight) can be explained by changes in X (daily calories consumed). These methods allow one to answer our third basic question: How much of the variation in weight is attributable to variation in daily calories consumed?

Linear regression methods can be extended to include a large number of variables. This extension is known as *multiple linear regression*. For instance, in addition to the relationship to daily calories consumed, one might want to study in individuals the relationship of current height, current skull thickness, and weight at birth as independent variables versus current weight as the dependent variable. One might want to determine whether these other factors help explain a greater part of the variation in weight than daily calories alone.

In multiple linear regression, the Bs reflect the strength of the linear relationship between each independent variable (height for instance) and the dependent variable (weight) with the value of each other variable held constant. Multiple linear regression can thus be regarded as a multiple adjustment technique since adjustment for multiple variables occurs simultaneously. Multiple regression equations can be expressed as follows:

$$Y = B_1 x_1 + B_2 x_2 + B_3 x_3 + B_4 x_4 + c$$

Y = current weight

X_1 = current daily calories consumed

X_2 = current height

X_3 = weight at birth

X_4 = current skull thickness

c = constant representing the value of weight if all the Xs are extrapolated or extended to zero

Multiple regression equations are being widely used in medical research. If properly used they are a very helpful approach. They allow the simultaneous measurement of the strength of the associations between study factors and outcomes while holding other factors constant. One then can directly compare the size of B_1, B_2, B_3, and B_4 to determine which has the strongest association with weight. Statistical significance tests are available to test the statistical significance of each B. Methods used in conjunction with multiple regression also allow one to determine how much of the variation in outcome can be explained after all the study factors have been taken into account. Thus, the methods of multiple regression answer all three basic study questions on a large number of relationships simultaneously.

The example chosen here uses weight—a continuous variable—as the dependent variable. *Linear regression* requires that the dependent variable be continuous. It also assumes that the relationship between the dependent variable and each independent variable is linear. When a linear relationship is not suspected or the dependent variable is not continuous, other regression techniques are available. *Logistic regression* is useful when the dependent variable has two possible values such as dead versus alive, or improved versus not improved. When the dependent variable consists of more than two categories, *discriminant analysis* is useful.

In addition to answering the basic three questions about association and simultaneously adjusting for multiple independent variables, regression equations allow one further step. They permit the assessment of how useful the associations are for predicting the dependent variable or outcome for individuals not included in the study.

In order to test the ability of the known associations to predict the outcome, the previously derived regression equation is used, then data are obtained from individuals not included in the study. Using the example, this data would include daily calories consumed, height, skull thickness, and weight at birth. These values are plugged into the regression equation and a predicted adult weight can be calculated. The predicted weight then can be compared to the actual weight for each individual to get an idea of how well the regression equation works for prediction. In other words, the Bs and the c are derived from the previous study and the Xs are obtained from a new sample. The observed Ys in the new sample then can be compared to the predicted Ys.

The ability to make accurate predictions might be regarded as the ultimate goal of studying associations. Unfortunately, in medicine it is rarely possible to accurately predict outcome on an individual basis. For example, consider the strong association between smoking and lung cancer, which has been demonstrated repeatedly to be statistically significant. Furthermore, for those individuals included in studies, most of the risk of lung cancer usually can be attributed to smoking. Despite the ability of this association to gain high marks on each of our study questions, when applied to individuals in the general population, smoking does not do a very good job of predicting which individuals will develop lung cancer. This is true despite the strong association between smoking and lung cancer, because most individuals who smoke do not develop lung cancer. This fact implies that there are additional factors that need to be elucidated before it will be possible to predict who will develop lung cancer.

Investigators are often tempted to rely exclusively on regression techniques because they are computerized and can handle multiple variables simultaneously. It is important, however, to look first at the study factors one by one in order to understand the basic relationships established in the data. Proper choice of which variables to include also requires a close inspection of the variables one at a time. Thus regression techniques do not replace the methods discussed in the previous chapters. They merely serve to build upon and thus supplement the analysis obtained using the other methods.

When confronted with a regression method, it is important to keep in mind the basic questions about associations. It is easy to get caught up in fancy statistical footwork and lose sight of the basic questions. Remember to start by looking at the size of the B values. These are sometimes called coefficients. Look next at the p values for each of the B values. Regardless of the complexity of a statistical procedure, the p value still asks the same question: What is the probability of obtaining the observed data if the null hypothesis is true?

Regression methods usually have an expression such as R^2, which directly answers the third basic question: How much of the variation in the dependent variable can be explained by the independent variables? Finally, it is important to understand why the authors have used a regression method: Was it used in order to perform adjustment for many variables simultaneously; to determine which variables are most important; or to determine how well a regression equation that is developed on one study group predicts the outcome in another group?

The questions statistical tests ask, the way to properly choose a statistical test, and the meaning of the results are summarized and put it into a flowsheet that will be useful for study or reference (Fig. 30-1; pp. 246–253).

The flowsheet can be used in two ways. The reader can start by looking at the type of question being asked and the type of data being used and can follow the flowsheet from the beginning. This will allow the reader to choose a statistical test to answer the question.

Alternatively, when reading an article the reviewer can see what statistical test has been used and then work backwards in the flowsheet to see what assumptions underlie the use of the test and what questions are being asked. The reader then can make an independent judgment regarding the appropriateness of the statistical techniques used.

To demonstrate the use of the flowsheet, imagine that a study was conducted comparing the effect of a new antihypertensive drug on the diastolic blood pressure of a study group sample in comparison to an unmatched control group sample given a placebo.

To use the flowsheet, we need to answer the following questions:

1. Are samples or entire populations being employed?
2. Are we interested in differences or associations?
3. Is the outcome or dependent variable composed of nominal, ordinal, or continuous data?
4. How many comparisons are being made?
5. Have the study and control group individuals been matched?

In this example we are using samples; we are interested in differences between the outcomes; the dependent variable—change in diastolic blood pressure—is a continuous variable; there are two groups or one comparison, and the groups are not matched.

To use the flowsheet start at the top and choose the box marked "Samples." Next, choose the division marked "Difference." The boxes under "Difference" indicate that we are interested in measuring the size of the difference as observed in the data as well as testing the statistical significance of the differences that have been found. To determine how to report the differences observed in the data, we follow the circled 1 to the next sheet. Since our data is continuous, the flowsheet indicates that the differences should be reported as a difference between the mean values as well as a standard deviation for each group.

To determine which statistical significance test to use, we then turn back to the first flowsheet. Statistical significance tests are divided into techniques for nominal, ordinal, and continuous data. Since we are using continuous data, we now turn to the flowsheet that begins with the circled 4. In choosing the proper statistical significance test, proceed to the box marked "One comparison." Finally, we choose the test for unmatched samples: the t test.

This procedure tells us that the t test is an appropriate technique for performing a statistical significance test on our data. Similar use of the flowsheet allows one to choose the appropriate measures for different types of data when associations are being investigated.

The flowsheet also can be used in reverse so that when reading a study that employs a statistical technique, one can decide whether the technique was appropriate. Imagine that Pearson's coefficient of determination (r^2) is used to measure how much of the variation in triglyceride levels can be explained by variation in cholesterol levels.

To use the flowsheet, one first searches the bottom of the pages and locates Pearson's coefficient of determination (r^2) in the bottom right-hand box on the last sheet. Moving up the flowsheet, one reaches the box containing "Continuous data when a linear relationship is suspected."

This box indicates that Pearson's coefficient of determination (r^2) is applicable when both the variables consist of continuous data and when a linear relationship exists between the variables. Cholesterol and triglycerides are both measured using continuous data. To test whether a linear relationship exists, one would graph the data placing triglycerides on one axis and cholesterol on the other. If the relationship appears linear, then Pearson's coefficient of determination would be an appropriate technique.

Proceeding further up this sheet, one comes to the circled 7. This refers the reader back to the first sheet. Above the circled 7 on the first sheet is a box containing "Extent association explains variation between groups." This box says that Pearson's coefficient of determination (r^2) answers one of our basic questions about association, which for this example means how much of the variation in triglycerides can be explained by variation in the cholesterol. Since this is the question we originally sought to answer, Pearson's coefficient of determination (r^2) is an appropriate measure.

The flowsheet can be used in a similar fashion for other statistical measures to help the reader appreciate whether a proper statistical measure is being used and what question is being addressed.

Now that you are ready to apply the techniques of analysis to an article, sit down with the article, the uniform frameworks, the checklists of questions to ask, and the flowsheet. Review the basic questions that each type of study attempts to answer. Don't be mesmerized by the statistics, and don't expect the research to be perfect. It is, after all, a human creation constrained by reality. Try to remember that errors in studies do not necessarily invalidate the research; many a milestone in medicine has resulted from a less than ideal study. With enough thoughtful practice, you will find that reading the medical literature can be a pleasure.

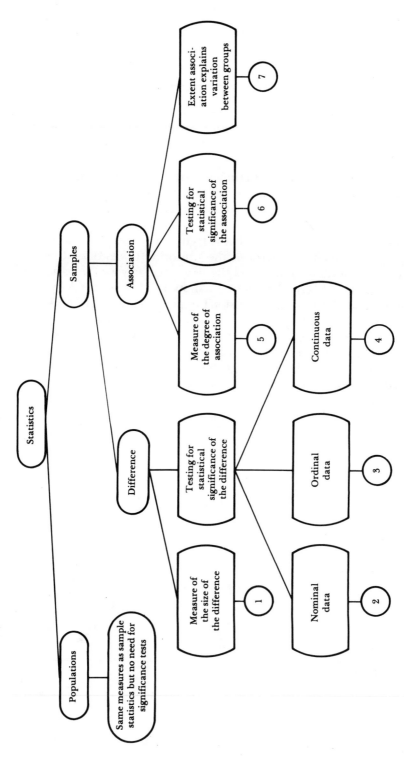

FIGURE 30-1. Flowsheet. In order to determine the correct statistical test to use for a given set of data, start at the beginning of the flowsheet. The numbers in circles indicate where to continue and are reproduced at the tops of the following pages (pp. 247–253). The numbers also are a guide for beginning with a specific test and working backwards.

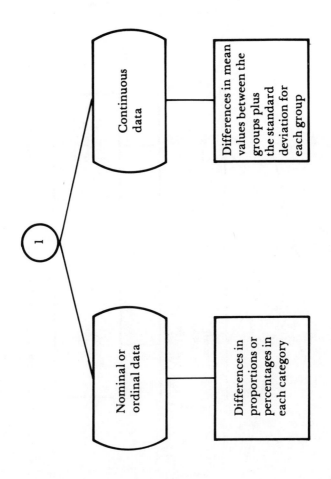

247

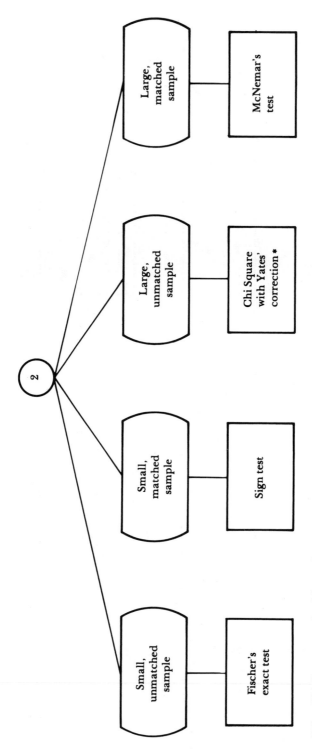

*The Chi Square method is used when comparing more than two groups. Yates' correction is used only when comparing two groups.

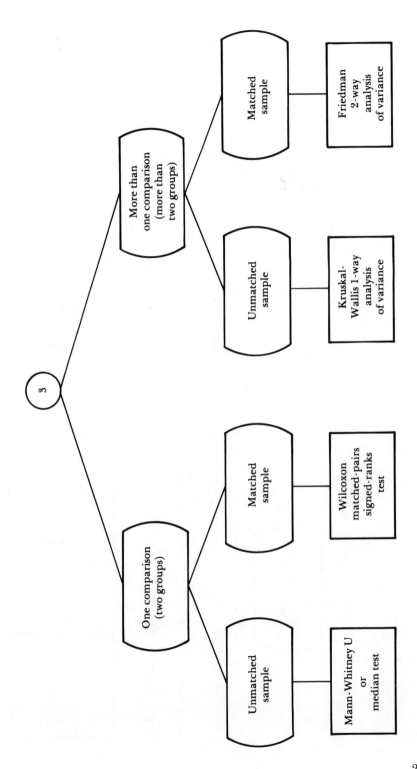

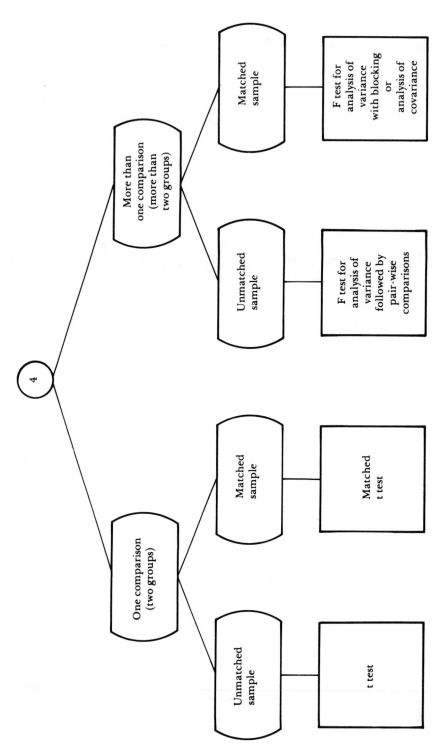

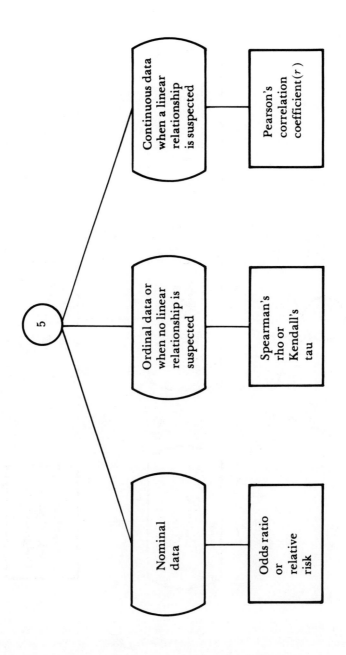

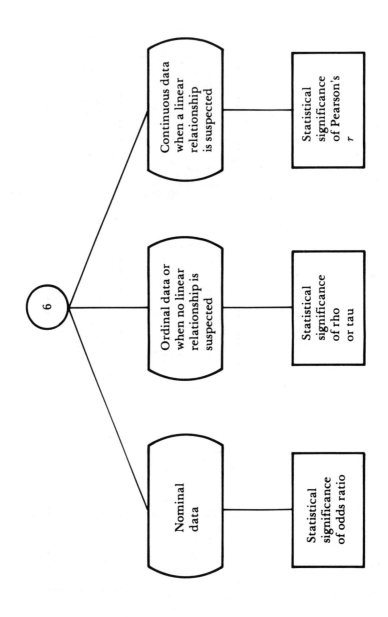

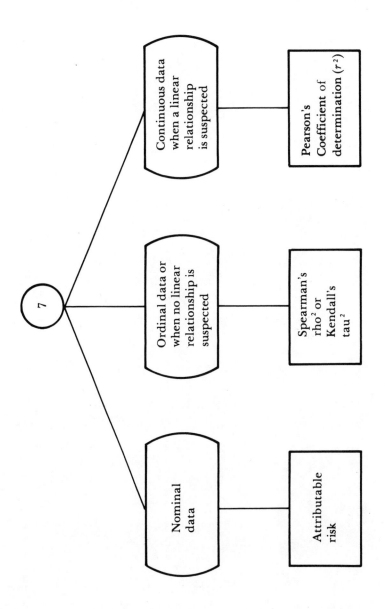

ADJUSTMENT Techniques used after the collection of data to take into account or control for the effects of known or potential confounding variables, that is, factors that differ both in the study and control groups that affect outcome.

ANALYSIS The comparison of the outcome of the study and control groups.

ARTIFACTUAL DIFFERENCES OR CHANGES Differences or changes in rates that result from the way the disease or condition is measured, sought, or defined.

ASSESSMENT The determination of the outcome of the study and control groups.

ASSIGNMENT The selection of individuals for study and control groups.

ASSOCIATION The occurrence together of two or more characteristics or events more often than would be expected by chance.

ATTRIBUTABLE RISK A measure of the proportion of the total risk that is explained by, or attributable to, the characteristic or risk factor under study.

BLIND ASSESSMENT The determination of the outcome for individuals without the person who makes the determination knowing whether the individuals were in the study group or the control group.

BLIND ASSIGNMENT Blind assignment occurs when individuals are assigned to a study group and a control group with neither the investigator nor the subjects being aware of the group to which they are assigned. When both investigator and subjects are "blinded," the study is sometimes referred to as a double-blind study.

CASE CONTROL *See* RETROSPECTIVE STUDY.

CHI SQUARE Statistical techniques used for nominal data which are applicable to one or more comparisons if the expected numbers are large enough. "Large enough" is generally defined as five or more.

CHUNK SAMPLE Use of only a portion of the total population of interest. Usually assembled because of the ease of collecting the data without regard for the degree to which the sample is random or representative of the population of interest.

CLINICAL STUDY A general term used to include retrospective, prospective, cross-sectional, and experimental studies performed on humans.

CLINICAL TRIAL *See* EXPERIMENTAL STUDY.

COHORT A group of individuals who share a common exposure or experience. Applies to prospective studies in which the study

255

group and the control group each share a common experience. Also applies to a cohort effect in which change in rates are explained by a unique experience shared by a subgroup of the population.

COHORT EFFECT A change in rates that can be explained by the unique experience of a group or cohort of individuals. A cohort effect implies that current rates should not be directly extrapolated into the future.

COHORT STUDY *See* PROSPECTIVE STUDY.

CONCURRENT PROSPECTIVE STUDY A prospective study in which an individual's assignment is determined at the time the study begins, and individuals are followed forward for the duration of the study.

CONFIDENCE LIMITS OF THE MEAN The range of possible values within which the parent population's mean is likely to fall. Confidence limits for a parent population are calculated using the mean, standard deviation, and size of the sample. A 95% confidence limit of the mean says that with 95% confidence one can say that the parent population's mean falls within this range.

CONFOUNDING VARIABLE A variable that differs between the study group and the control group, affecting the outcome being assessed.

CONTINUOUS DATA A type of data in which there is an unlimited number of equally spaced categories. Continuous data do not imply that there is unlimited variation among human populations.

CONTRIBUTORY CAUSE The characteristic referred to as the cause precedes the effect; by altering the cause the effect is also altered.

CONTROL GROUP A population or sample of a population that is used for comparison with a study group. Ideally, the control group is identical to the study group except that it does not possess the characteristic or has not been exposed to the treatment under study.

CROSS-SECTIONAL STUDY A study that begins by identifying individuals with and without the condition or disease under study. It then compares them to determine the proportion of each group that currently possesses a characteristic or is currently being exposed to a factor.

DEPENDENT VARIABLE Originally used in experimental studies to designate the characteristic under study to determine how it varied with changes made by the investigator in the independent variable. As used here, it refers more generally to the outcome variable in any type of research study.

DISCRIMINANT ANALYSIS A regression technique that is useful when the dependent variable consists of more than two categories of possible outcomes.

ECOLOGICAL FALLACY Error committed by investigators who extrapolate from general population data to the individuals within that population, without determining whether the relationship established by comparing populations actually holds for individuals.

EFFECT An outcome that is brought about, at least in part, by an etiological factor known as the cause.

EFFECT OF OBSERVATION Threat to validity that results when the process of observation alters the outcome of the study.

EXPERIMENTAL ACCURACY Precision of a test when applied under strictly controlled conditions.

EXPERIMENTAL STUDY (OR CLINICAL TRIAL) A study in which the investigator assigns individuals to both a study and a control group prior to the occurrence of the study condition or outcome. Only experimental studies allow random and blind assignment of individuals to study and control groups.

EXTRAPOLATION Conclusions drawn about the meaning of the study for the larger population not included in the study.

FALSE NEGATIVE When an individual's value on a test is negative but the disease or condition is present as determined by the gold standard, then the test has produced a false negative.

FALSE POSITIVE When an individual's value on a test is positive but the disease or condition is absent as determined by the gold standard, then the test has produced a false positive.

FIELD ACCURACY The precision of a test when applied under real clinical conditions.

GOLD STANDARD The criteria used to unequivically define the presence of a condition or disease under study.

HYPOTHESIS The assertion that an association between two or more variables or a difference between two or more groups exists in the larger population of interest.

INCIDENCE RATE An approximation of the risk of developing a given disease. Calculated by taking the ratio of the number of individuals who develop the condition over a period of time, divided by the number of individuals in the population at the midpoint of the time interval.

INDEPENDENT VARIABLE   Originally used in experimental studies to designate the factor or variable being manipulated by the investigator. As used here, it refers to the variable or factor being studied in order to determine the effects on the outcome or dependent variable in any type of research study.

INHERENT SAMPLING ERROR   An error introduced by chance differences between the results obtained in a sample and the true value in the larger population from which the sample was drawn. Sampling error is present even in randomly obtained samples. It is inherent in the use of sampling methods.

INSTRUMENT ERROR   A threat to the precision of assessment that results when the testing instrument is not suited to the conditions of the study or is not precise enough in measuring the study outcome.

INTEROBSERVER VARIATION   Variation in results or outcomes brought about by differences in interpretation by different individuals.

INTERPRETATION   The drawing of conclusions about the meaning of any differences found between the study group and the control group for those included in the investigation.

INTRAOBSERVER VARIATION   Variation in results or outcome resulting from differences in interpretations by the same person at different times.

LINEAR CORRELATION METHODS   Statistical methods used for studying the degree and statistical significance of an association when a straight line relationship exists between the variables being investigated.

LINEAR REGRESSION   Statistical methods used to study the relationship between independent and dependent variables when the dependent variable consists of continuous data.

LOGISTIC REGRESSION   A regression technique that is useful when the dependent variable consists of two categories of possible outcomes.

MATCHING (*See also* PAIRING)   A procedure used at the beginning of studies that selects control individuals who possess the same characteristic as study individuals. Matching is done to control for a confounding variable and to reduce the number of individuals required for a study.

MEAN   Sum of the values divided by the number of entities or individuals. A statistical term for the average.

NECESSARY CAUSE The characteristic referred to as the cause is always found in the presence of the effect.

NOMINAL DATA A type of data in which there are a limited number of categories but no inherent ordering of the categories.

NONCONCURRENT PROSPECTIVE STUDY A prospective study in which an individual's assignment is determined prior to the time the study begins, but before the time of occurrence of the outcome under study. Individuals then are followed forward in time to assess the development of the outcome under study.

NONPARAMETRIC STATISTICS Nonparametric statistics are applicable especially to ordinal data. They can also be used when the assumptions necessary for the use of other techniques are not fulfilled.

NORMAL DISTRIBUTION An important distribution in statistics, the shape approximates a bell-shaped curve. The normal distribution is symmetrical, continuous, and has a mean value that lies at the highest point on the curve.

NULL HYPOTHESIS The assertion that no true difference between groups or association between study characteristics exists in the larger parent population.

ODDS RATIO The odds ratio is a measure of the degree or strength of an association applicable to all types of studies employing nominal data, but usually applied to retrospective and cross-sectional studies. The odds ratio for retrospective and cross-sectional studies is measured as the odds of having the risk factor if the condition is present, divided by the odds of having the risk factor if the condition is not present.

ONE-TAILED TEST A modification of a statistical significance test in which differences or associations in only the direction predicted by the hypothesis are considered. Use of a one-tailed test implies that the investigator would not be interested in differences or associations if they had occurred in the opposite direction.

ORDINAL DATA A type of data in which there is a limited number of categories with an inherent ordering of the categories from lowest to highest. Ordinal data however says nothing about the spacing between categories.

PAIRING A special form of matching in which each study individual is coupled or paired with a control individual and their outcome data are compared. When pairing is used, special statistical methods should be employed in the analysis that take advantage of the ability of pairing to increase the statistical power of the study. Statistical significance tests for "matching" actually refer to pairing.

PAIR-WISE COMPARISONS   A comparison between two groups that aims to determine which comparison contributes to the overall statistical significance. Pair-wise comparisons are performed after having first demonstrated an overall statistical significance using the data from all groups together.

PARAMETER   The value from the larger parent population that is estimated by a statistic derived from a sample of the parent population.

PARENT POPULATION   The entire larger population or population of interest from which a sample is obtained. The parent population includes all those to whom the investigators would like to extrapolate their results.

PEARSON'S CORRELATION COEFFICIENT (r)   A measure of degree of association that assumes a linear relationship between the variables and continuous data for each of the variables. The value of r varies from $+1$ to -1.

PEARSON'S COEFFICIENT OF DETERMINATION (r^2)   The square of the sample correlation coefficient r. Indicates the proportion of the variation in one variable that is explained by variation in the other.

PLACEBO   Inert or ineffectual substance given to control individuals in an experimental study to remove or reduce the possibility that the subject's belief in treatment can itself alter the outcome.

POPULATION STATISTICS   Statistical techniques used when the entire population of interest is included in a study. These techniques are the same as when samples are used except that there is no need for statistical significance tests.

POWER OF A STATISTICAL SIGNIFICANCE TEST   The ability of the test to detect a statistically significant difference or association in sample data if a true difference or association is present in the larger parent populations.

PREDICTIVE VALUE OF A NEGATIVE TEST   The proportion of those with a negative test who actually do not have the condition or disease as measured by the gold standard. This measure incorporates the prevalence of the condition or disease. Clinically, the predictive value of a negative test is the probability that an individual is free of the disease if the test is negative.

PREDICTIVE VALUE OF A POSITIVE TEST   The proportion of those with a positive test who actually have the condition or disease as measured by the gold standard. This measure incorporates the prevalence of the condition or disease. Clinically, the predictive value of a positive test is the probability that an individual has the disease if the test is positive.

PREVALENCE   An approximation of the risk of having a given disease at a given point in time. The prevalence rate is calculated by taking the ratio of those who have the condition at a point in time divided by the number of individuals in the population at the same point in time. As used in diagnostic tests, the prevalence refers to the probability of the disease being present before the test is performed. Prevalence in this sense also is called *pretest probability* or *prior probability.*

PROSPECTIVE STUDY (OR COHORT STUDY)   A study in which a group classified by the presence or absence of a factor is followed to determine whether those with the factor have a greater or lesser likelihood of developing the disease or condition under study. Prospective studies can be done concurrently or nonconcurrently.

RANDOM ASSIGNMENT (OR RANDOMIZATION)   Individuals chosen for the study have equal chance of being assigned either to the study group or to the control group. Random assignment is only possible in an experimental study. Randomization does not assure that the study group or the control group will be identical with respect to all characteristics that affect the outcome of an investigation.

RANDOM SAMPLE   A sample in which each individual or entity in the larger population of interest has an equal opportunity of being included in the sample. Statistical significance testing requires that the study group and the control group each be random samples of all those who could have been selected. It does not require randomization.

RANGE OF NORMAL   A range of values in a test that usually includes 95% of the individuals who are free of disease.

RATE   An approximation of risk calculated as a ratio of the times the event occurs divided by the number of individuals in the population at a point in time.

RECALL ERROR   Threat to the precision of assessment that results when subjects in one of the groups being compared are more accurate in remembering past events than subjects in other groups.

REGRESSION TECHNIQUES   A series of statistical methods that are useful for studying the association between one dependent variable and many independent variables. Regression techniques are capable of measuring the degree of association, the statistical significance of an association, and the extent that the association explains the variation in outcome. Regression techniques are also useful for performing multiple simultaneous adjustments and serving as a basis for prediction.

REGRESSION TO THE MEAN   A principle stating that unusual events are unlikely to recur. By chance alone, events subsequent to an unusual event are likely to be closer to the average.

RELATIVE RISK   The probability of developing the outcome if the risk factor is present divided by the probability of developing the outcome if the risk factor is not present. The relative risk is a measure of the strength or degree of association applicable to prospective and experimental studies. In retrospective and cross-sectional studies the odds ratio is used to approximate the relative risk.

REPORTING ERROR   Threat to the precision of assessment that results when the subjects in one of the groups are more apt to accurately report previous events than members of other groups being compared.

REPRODUCIBILITY   The ability of a test to produce consistent results when independently repeated and interpreted under nearly identical circumstances.

RETROSPECTIVE STUDY (OR CASE CONTROL)   A study that begins by identifying cases and controls and compares them to determine the proportion of each group that previously possessed a characteristic or an exposure to a factor.

RISK FACTOR   An individual characteristic or factor that has been shown to be associated with an increased odds ratio or relative risk of developing a condition or disease. A risk factor does not necessarily imply cause and effect. There is often ambiguity in use of the term *risk factor*. It may or may not imply that the risk factor precedes the development of the condition or disease.

RISK OF OCCURRENCE   Probability of developing a given disease or condition as measured by the number of cases occurring over a period of time divided by the number of individuals in the population during the same period of time. This measure is known as absolute risk in contrast to relative risk that compares the risk to those exposed to or possessing a study factor versus those who do not.

SAMPLE A subset of a larger population obtained for investigation in order to draw conclusions about the larger parent population.

SAMPLE STATISTICS Statistical techniques used when studies are performed on samples of a larger population of interest. Statistical significance tests are then necessary to relate findings in the samples to those of the larger populations of interest.

SELECTION BIAS An error in assignment that occurs whenever the selection of study and control individuals produces a difference between the groups that affects the results of the study.

SENSITIVITY The proportion of those with the disease or condition as measured by the gold standard who are positive by the test being studied.

SPECIFICITY The proportion of those without the disease or condition as measured by the gold standard who are negative by the test being studied.

STANDARD DEVIATION A commonly used measure of the spread or variation within a sample composed of continuous data. The standard deviation measures the variation of the data itself.

STANDARD ERROR OF THE MEAN A measure derived from a sample's standard deviation and sample size that attempts to relate the observed mean obtained in the data to the true mean of the larger population of interest.

STANDARDIZATION (OF A RATE) An effort to take into account or adjust for the effects of a factor such as age or sex on the obtained rates.

STATISTIC A summary measure derived from sample data that is used to estimate a value in the larger parent population.

STATISTICAL SIGNIFICANCE TEST Statistical technique for determining the probability that the observed or larger differences or associations would occur by chance alone if there is no true difference or association in the larger parent population.

STRATIFIED RANDOM SAMPLE A sample in which the population is first divided into parts, known as strata, and a random sample obtained from each of the strata.

STUDY GROUP In a prospective or experimental study, a group of individuals who possess the characteristics or are exposed to the factors under study. In a retrospective or cross-sectional study, a group of individuals who have developed the disease or condition being investigated.

SUFFICIENT CAUSE   The characteristic referred to as the effect is always found in the presence of the characteristic referred to as the cause.

TRUE NEGATIVE   A true negative indicates that the individual did not have the disease or condition as measured by either the gold standard or the test being studied.

TRUE POSITIVE   A true positive indicates that the individual had the disease or condition as measured by both the gold standard and the test being studied.

TWO-TAILED TEST   A modification of a statistical significance test in which a difference or association in both the direction of the hypothesis and in the opposite direction are considered. Use of a two-tailed test implies that the investigator would be interested in differences or associations if they had occurred in the opposite direction. When in doubt a two-tailed test is preferable.

TYPE I ERROR   An error that occurs when using data from samples that demonstrates a statistically significant difference or association when no true difference or association exists in the parent populations.

TYPE II ERROR   An error that occurs from failure to demonstrate a statistically significant difference or association in sample data when one actually exists in the larger parent populations.

VALIDITY   The extent to which a study or test measures what it purports to measure.

VARIABLE   A characteristic of an individual, an object, or an event that can be classified or measured. *See also* DEPENDENT VARIABLE and INDEPENDENT VARIABLE.

Selected Readings

Bahn, A. K. *Basic Medical Statistics.* New York: Grune & Stratton, 1972.

Brown, B. W. *Statistics: A Biomedical Introduction.* New York: Wiley, 1977.

Campbell, D. T., and Stanley, J. C. *Experimental and Quasi-Experimental Designs for Research.* Chicago: Rand McNally, 1963.

Cochran, W. G., and Snedecor, G. W. *Statistical Methods* (7th ed.). Ames, Iowa: Iowa State University Press, 1980.

Colton, T. *Statistics in Medicine.* Boston: Little, Brown, 1974.

Conover, W. J. *Practical Nonparametric Statistics* (2nd ed). New York: Wiley, 1980.

Feinstein, A. R. *Clinical Biostatistics.* St. Louis: Mosby, 1977.

Fleiss, J. L. *Statistical Methods for Rates and Proportions.* New York: Wiley, 1973.

Griner, P. F. et al. Selection and interpretation of diagnostic tests and procedures. *Ann. Intern. Med.* 94:553, 1981.

Haach, D. G. *Statistical Literacy: A Guide to Interpretation.* North Scituate, Massachusetts: Duxbury Press, 1979.

Hill, A. B. *Principles of Medical Statistics* (9th ed.). London: Lancet, 1971.

Huff, D. *How to Lie with Statistics.* New York: Norton, 1954.

Hutchison, G. B., and Shapiro, S. Lead time gained by diagnostic screening for breast cancer. *J.N.C.I.* 41:665, 1968.

Lilienfeld, A. M. Some limitations and problems of screening for cancer. *Cancer* 33:1720, 1974.

Lilienfeld, A. M. *Foundations of Epidemiology.* New York: Oxford University Press, 1976.

Lilienfeld, A. M., et al. *Cancer Epidemiology: Methods of Study.* Baltimore: Johns Hopkins Press, 1967.

Linton, M. *The Practical Statistician: Simplified Handbook of Statistics.* Monterey, California: Brooks/Cole Pub. Co., 1975.

MacMahon, B. and Pugh, T. F. *Epidemiology Principles and Methods.* Boston: Little, Brown, 1970.

Mausner, J. S., and Bahn, A. K. *Epidemiology: An Introductory Text.* Philadelphia: Saunders, 1974.

Murphy, E. A. *The Logic of Medicine.* Baltimore: Johns Hopkins Press, 1976.

Murphy, E. A. *Probability in Medicine.* Baltimore: Johns Hopkins Press, 1979.

Siegel, S. *Nonparametric Statistics for the Behavioral Sciences.* New York: McGraw-Hill, 1956.

Susser, M. *Causal Thinking in the Health Sciences. Concepts and Strategies in Epidemiology.* New York: Oxford University Press, 1973.

Swinscow, T. D. V. *Statistics at Square One.* London: British Medical Association, 1976.

Williams, F. *Reasoning with Statistics* (2nd ed.). New York: Holt, Rinehart and Winston, 1979.

Wilson, J. G., and Jungner, F. Principles and Practice of Screening for Disease. Public Health Papers No. 34, WHO, Geneva, 1968.

Index

Index

Absolute risk, defined, 225
Accuracy of diagnostic tests. *See*
 Diagnostic tests, accuracy of
Accuracy of sampling. *See*
 Samples/sampling, accuracy of
Adjustment
 of data. *See* Data, adjustment of
 of range of normal in tests,
 104–105, 106, 111–113, 139
 false negatives/false positives and,
 105, 106
 of rates, defined, 167. *See also*
 Standardization of rates
Aims of study, adequate definition of,
 63, 71, 73
Analysis, 29–41
 of clinical trials, 11, 13, 85
 confounding variables and, 29–30,
 72, 73
 defined, 7, 8
 evaluation of, 72
 flaw-catching exercises, 77–79, 81,
 85, 88–90
 prior matching of individual and
 control groups and, 30–31
 prospective studies, 7, 12, 81, 88–90
 questions on, 73–74
 retrospective studies, 9, 10, 77–79
 statistical significance testing, 31–41,
 72, 73, 74. *See also* Statistical
 significance test(s)
Artifactual changes/differences in
 rates. *See* Rate(s), artifactual
 changes in
Assessment of outcome, 21–27
 appropriate measures of, 21–22, 71,
 73
 criteria for, 21–22
 blind, 24
 completeness of, 25–26
 criteria for valid measures of, 21–27
 defined, 7, 8
 evaluation, 71
 experimental studies, 11, 13, 84–85
 flaw-catching exercises, 77, 84–85,
 88
 imprecise measurement/instrument
 error, 22, 24

incomplete follow-up, 25–26
investigative errors/
 misinterpretation, 24–25
observational process and, 21,
 26–27, 71, 73
precise, 21, 22–25
prospective studies, 11, 12,
 81, 88
questions on, 73
recall errors, 22–23
reporting errors, 23–24
reports by individuals and, 22–24
retrospective studies, 9, 10, 77
Assignment, 15–19
 blind, 11
 chance and, 19
 comparability and, 18–19, 71, 73
 defined, 7, 8
 double-blind, 11
 evaluation, 71
 in experimental studies, 11, 13, 84
 flaw-catching exercises, 80–81, 84,
 87, 88
 in prospective studies, 9, 12, 80–81,
 87, 88
 questions on, 73
 random, 11, 19
 in retrospective studies, 9, 10, 77
 selection bias and, 19, 71, 73
Association(s), 206, 207, 223–237,
 237–242
 cause and effect and, 223
 degree/strength, 224
 regression methods in
 measurement, 237, 238
 dependent variable in
 defined, 223
 variation, independent variable
 variation and, 237, 239,
 241–242
 example of demonstration of,
 223–224
 implications of, 223
 independent variable in, defined,
 223
 nominal data, 224–231
 in prospective/experimental
 studies, 224–228, 232, 235

269